T0065721

staying fit
after
forty

A Plan for Healthy & Active Living

staying fit after forty

Don S. Otis, editor

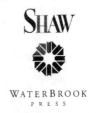

SHAW

WATERBROOK
PRESS

Staying Fit After Forty
A SHAW BOOK
PUBLISHED BY WATERBROOK PRESS
2375 Telstar Drive, Suite 160
Colorado Springs, Colorado 80920
A division of Random House, Inc.

All Scripture quotations, unless otherwise indicated, are taken from the *Holy Bible, New International Version®*. NIV® Copyright © 1973, 1978, 1984 by International Bible Society. Used by permission of Zondervan Publishing House. All rights reserved. Scripture quotations marked (Phillips) are taken from *The New Testament in Modern English, Revised Edition* © 1972 by J. B. Phillips. Scripture quotations marked (RSV) are taken from the *Revised Standard Version of the Bible*, copyright © 1946, 1952, and 1971 by the Division of Christian Education of the National Council of the Churches of Christ in the USA. Used by permission. Scripture quotations marked (KJV) are taken from the *King James Version*.

ISBN 978-0-877-88453-8

Library of Congress Cataloging-in-Publication Data
Staying fit after forty : a plan for healthy and active living / [edited by] Don S. Otis.
    p.   cm.
    "A Shaw book."
    ISBN 9780877884538(pbk.)
        1. Physical fitness for middle aged persons.   2. Exercise for middle aged persons.
    3. Middle aged persons—Health and hygiene.   4. Aging.   I. Otis, Don S., 1956–

RA777.5 .S73   2001
613.7'044—dc21

                                                  00-053186

Printed in the United States of America
2001—First Shaw Edition

146502721

Contents

Acknowledgments

As a young teenager, I was grateful for parents who hauled me to community track meets, Little League games, and nearby mountains. My love for sports began at home, and it has never ended. Even today, with so many distractions from entertainment and technology, I would prefer to participate in physical activities than to be a detached viewer. Vicarious thrills never interested me much. I have always wanted to be on the experiential end. Still, this book could not have been done effectively on my own knowledge or life experiences. Instead, it weaves the collective ideas, experiences, and wisdom of some of the finest practitioners I know.

I deeply appreciate those who have contributed their time and expertise. Because of their efforts, this book is a valuable tool for extending our life and ministry to others. My sincerest appreciation extends to Dr. Andrew Seddon of Billings, Montana; Judy Lindberg McFarland of Palos Verdes, California; Dr. Mary Ruth Swope of Avinger, Texas; Dr. Gregory Jantz of Seattle, Washington; Maryanna Young of Fitness Management Group in Boise, Idaho; Pastor Jeff Mitchum of San Diego, California; Tom Mason of Colorado Springs, Colorado; and Laurie Ellsworth of Champaign, Illinois.

There are also numerous people who gave the time to share their secrets for success in fitness and life. They are the success stories—those who lend credibility through their experiences. Many of these stories came from people I see every week at one of the finest fitness facilities in the Northwest—Sandpoint West Athletic Club.

I am thankful to Joan Guest, who saw the potential in this project. Additional thanks to those at Shaw/WaterBrook Press who helped make this possible—Dan Rich, Don Pape, Elisa Fryling, and Carol Bartley.

Introduction

Exercise is the most effective anti-aging pill ever discovered.

—NATIONAL INSTITUTES OF HEALTH

John A. Kelley is the quintessential workhorse of the Boston Marathon. At ninety-two years old, Kelley just keeps moving. He has run the Boston Marathon dozens of time, even winning it on occasion. Unlike the mythical unicorn that serves as the mascot for the Boston Athletic Association, Kelley is every bit flesh and blood. I wondered what kept this man going year in and year out. My curiosity was similar to the befuddled reporter who asked the British climber George Mallory why he wanted to summit Mount Everest. What his answer lacked in erudition, it made up for in conciseness: "Because it is there!"

I approached the aged John Kelley in Boston to ask him a couple of questions, hoping he would oblige me with some insight into his passion for running. "What advice do you have for people who are getting older?" I queried Kelley. He shot back, "Keep moving. Do whatever you can to stay active. Find something you like to do and then do it!"

It is obvious that this exercise veteran has followed his own advice. Although he has lived nearly two decades beyond the average American male, he continues to add to the tens of thousands of miles he has already logged. His mind is clear and sharp, and his body fit and trim.

While many of us may never live to be ninety, statistics show that more Americans expect to live longer than current life-expectancy projections. Yet America ranks twenty-fourth in the world for life expectancy. This is deplorable for a country with such sophisticated medical facilities and treatment options. The problem? Americans continue to indulge in high-fat diets and are simply not getting the activity they need to stay healthy as they age.

As we get older, our thinking naturally shifts to ways we can live healthier lives. We want to know how we can remain independent well into our senior years. This is not an impossibility. Gerontologists are now starting to refer to a measurement called "functional age" to describe our physical abilities as we get older. Of course, lifestyle choices contribute greatly to how we age. Still, people who regularly exercise have a functional age much lower than that of their peers who do not exercise regularly.[1]

So is it simply a matter of deciding to start exercising—and then doing it? Not exactly. Like preparing for a successful financial retirement, we need a plan. Without one, much of our investment of time and energy is likely to be wasted. This book will provide more than a plan: It will offer help in nutrition, motivation, weight control, injuries, and serious exercise. You will read real-life examples of people who have struggled with the same issues you face—not just theories from twenty-something bodybuilders. You will hear from everyday practitioners, people who know what it's like to have aches and pains, stiff joints, injuries, and hectic lifestyles.

Potluck Christianity

While there are plenty of good reasons to take care of the "temple" God has given each of us, the church, surprisingly, has not always encouraged us to remain active and eat healthfully. In fact, chances are that in most church bulletins you are far more likely to find an invitation to a potluck picnic than an aerobics class. According to recent research from Purdue University, religious people tend to be more corpulent than nonreligious people. The more religious you are, the fatter you tend to be! At the same time, actively practicing one's religion is the most consistent predictor of overall well-being in our culture.[2]

While most Christians traditionally have avoided such self-destructive activities as smoking or drinking heavily, we have not led the way in either fitness or nutrition. Instead, New Age adherents and followers of Eastern religions seem to have done a better job of embracing good nutrition. They have integrated it into their lifestyles and religious observances. And though some Christians participate in sports or physical activities, this is not because it has been emphasized in the church.

We wrongly see obesity or poor eating habits as lesser evils than drinking or smoking. In reality, they are no less destructive to our bodies. "The evidence is now compelling and irrefutable," says JoAnn Manson of Harvard University. "Obesity is probably the second-leading preventable cause of death in the United States after cigarette smoking."[3] Just twenty years ago, one-quarter of the U.S. population were considered obese. Today, one-third of all Americans are obese. Christian medical doctor and author Don Colbert says, "Even though most Americans have listened to the latest scientific research showing the perils of fats, sugar and high cholesterol, dangerous foods and a sedentary lifestyle, there is still a rise in obesity."[4]

According to the Centers for Disease Control, half of all overweight people are trying to lose weight. Meanwhile, the government is telling us that we are not exercising enough. Even former Health and Human Services Secretary Donna Shalala called this loss of physical education a national tragedy.[5] Yet most senior high schools have cut back their requirements for physical education! The minimum government recommendation for exercise is a mere thirty minutes a day, five days a week—just two and a half hours a week. And yet only about 15 percent of all Americans do this.

Somewhere along the way, the church got the idea that fitness and nutrition were unimportant or at least irrelevant to our faith. Perhaps it was the apostle Paul's claim that bodily exercise profits little (which we will discuss later) that influenced us to view exercise as a waste of time. After all, some of us reason it is the eternal things that really matter—the need for salvation and inner peace. Of course, there is an element of truth to these arguments. Yet health and fitness certainly play an indirect role in our ability to carry out the mandate and demands of the gospel. Anemic, overweight, poorly conditioned, or bedridden Christians have little or no energy for the work of the kingdom.

A Connection Between Faith and Health?

There is increasing evidence of a link between our faith and better health. A recent study at Duke University Medical Center found that people with strong religious beliefs recover faster from depression, have lower blood pressure, and have better-functioning immune systems than people who express no such beliefs. The difference in mortality rates between churchgoers and nonchurchgoers is as strong as the difference in mortality rates between smokers and nonsmokers.[6] What can we conclude from the Duke study? Generally, a belief in God gives us a purpose or meaning in life. It provides us with a set of reasonable rules to live by, rules that help us take better care of the equipment God has given us.

Study after study reveals that a strong sense of spirituality keeps people alive longer, keeps their marriages stronger, and keeps them mentally balanced, off drugs, out of jail, and out of hospitals. More than two hundred studies show a robust relationship between people who are more spiritually or religiously involved and the positive indicators of health.[7]

True Christianity includes the practice of forgiveness, rules to live by, prayer and meditation, inner peace, community, and avoidance of harmful habits. These practices all contribute to the general health of Christians. In fact, faith is so important that even when we do get sick or injured it helps in the recovery process. In a study of 542 patients, the average length of stay in the hospital for deeply religious people over sixty years of age was eleven days, compared with twenty-five days for nonreligious people.[8] In the long haul, there is no separation between our health and our faith.

Making Lifestyle Changes

Perhaps you picked up this book because you hope that it will change you in some miraculous way. I wish I could make that promise. But, frankly, this book is merely a tool that can help you make changes in your own life. It is designed to encourage you, inform you, and give you the nudge you may need to make the changes *on your own*. No one else can do it for you.

You might be surprised to learn that 68 percent of doctors nationwide have not exercised in the last year.[9] You would probably not be surprised, however, to learn that more than half of all Americans are overweight and that 20 percent are considered dangerously obese.[10] The sad irony is that if you asked a doctor if she should exercise, the chances are fairly good that she would say, "Absolutely!" And the chances are also fairly good that if you asked most overweight Americans if they would like to lose weight, they would also say, "Absolutely!" So why do we believe one way and habitually act another? Why don't we make the changes we know are good for us?

There is no one answer to this dilemma. If you have struggled with weight control or with maintaining an exercise routine, only you know the answers for your personal struggle. The one answer we can provide in this book, however, is how to help you find the strength to make the necessary personal changes and stick with them! Be assured that you are not alone. Many Americans want help with taking care of their bodies. But if you are one of the millions of people who want to change, read the information in each of these chapters, and apply it to your life *now*.

What You Will Learn

In the following pages, you will learn from people of all ages beyond forty who have put into practice what they have written about. Each of these people is a committed Christian who understands that serving Christ and honoring the people around us are what faith is about. They also understand that honoring God with body, mind, and spirit is a worthy task.

To help you accomplish your goals, we will cover a wide range of topics:

- how to get started and what you need to know about exercise
- how to overcome the obstacles to motivation
- what to do when you are injured
- how to fit exercise into a busy life
- ways to remain active after you retire
- what vitamins or supplements you should take and why
- how to eat right for weight control
- how to sustain long-term interest in exercise
- overcoming fear and past failures
- the Ten Commandments for Fitness
- serious exercise for those over forty

We have, to the best of our abilities and experiences, compiled a book that I am certain will benefit you for years to come if you apply its collective wisdom. Enjoy the journey!

ONE

Busy Lives: Finding Time for Fitness

DON OTIS

*I burn the candle on both ends, and I have at least five full-time jobs.
There is no way I could do that if I didn't keep myself in shape.*

—DR. KENNETH COOPER

Imagine what it was like in ancient Palestine. The roads were nothing more than dusty caravan routes in the summer. In the winter, they were mud bogs. These so-called roads were littered with debris and filth. It was not a pretty sight. Thousands of camels and donkeys used these routes to and from Jerusalem or on the way to Damascus. As was their custom, Jesus and His disciples walked these roads as well. That's how most people traveled—by foot. It was slow. And most carried their provisions strapped to their backs.

The Bible has little to say about exercise, because people in biblical times got their exercise by virtue of their lifestyle. Today we live in a different world. When it's hot or humid, we go from our air-conditioned houses to our air-conditioned cars to get to our air-conditioned offices. When we arrive at work, we sit in padded chairs. In our living rooms, we enjoy soft couches or overstuffed chairs.

How many times have you seen people fighting over a parking place at a crowded mall or grocery store, sometimes choosing to wait several minutes for a spot close to the stores? Today, if we have to park a hundred yards from a mall entrance, we think it's too crowded! Modern conveniences—microwave ovens, computers, cars, motorized lawn mowers, power tools, washers and dryers— make our lives easier. They replace activities that people just one hundred years ago were accustomed to doing as part of their everyday lives. Now we take these conveniences for granted. But while they certainly reduce the drudgery of certain kinds of work, they also reduce the need for physical labor to accomplish a day's work. In return, modern conveniences give us more free time than past generations had.

Few of us use our leisure time in activities that provide any meaningful physical benefits. Instead, too many spend far too much time in sedentary leisure—television, movies, or computer games. Others, however, do engage in sports or exercise. Still, it seems a bit ironic that we create new gadgets and technologies so we will have more time to go to the gym, golf, swim, or hike, yet so few of us take physical advantage of our new freedoms. We are clearly not prepared to give up air-conditioners, cars, or dishwashers anytime soon.

The challenge each of us faces today is to make a conscious effort to engage in physical activity that will benefit us. This chapter looks at how we can find time to stay active in the midst of a demanding schedule. It takes commitment. It takes intention. Only then will it become a habit. It is not impossible—though it may be a challenge—to remain active even with a busy schedule.

In this chapter I have enlisted the help of two seasoned fitness veterans. Dr. Gregory Jantz is a clinical therapist, speaker, and runner in his forties who provides thoughts about how to bring continuity between our bodies and spirits. Tom Mason is in his fifties and serves as a vice president at Focus on the Family. He explains how he finds time for fitness in spite of an extremely demanding schedule. First, however, let's look at some of the reasons or excuses for our busyness and ways we can respond to each demand on our time and energy.

Answering Our Busy-Life Excuses

Do any of the following too-busy-to-exercise comments sound familiar?

1. *"My children come first in my life. If I add exercise to an already busy schedule, they will suffer."* No one who has ever been a parent will argue with the fact that children are demanding on our time. When my kids were smaller, I would have them ride their bikes along next to me on what they unaffectionately referred to as a "bike-run-ride." Sometimes I would go to a high school running track and bring them with me. Once in a while they would run. Other times they played in the sand of the long-jump pit. They also enjoyed looking under the bleachers for money, water bottles, or other items of dubious value. After I finished running, we often threw a football or Frisbee. Instead of cutting into quality time with them, my exercise actually added to it.

2. *"My job takes me all over the country. It is simply too difficult to fit in exercise while I am traveling."* Sixty-year-old Texas businessman George McGough travels one hundred thousand miles every year. He says, "The most important thing I pack is my running

shoes…[Regular exercise is] a part of my life. It helps me live better." I admit, however, that exercise and travel don't mix well. All of us get into routines at home. When these routines are altered or disrupted, it is easier to do nothing. If you travel frequently, try to stay in hotels that have exercise facilities. Call ahead or check with your travel agent in advance.

Running or walking in new cities can be exhilarating. Or it can be downright frightening. Some big cities are safer than others. Ask at the front desk of your hotel before you venture out. Ask about the safest routes to parks or to streets with less traffic to contend with. Or get your workout without ever leaving the premises. On a recent trip to Florida, I had exactly forty-five minutes between the time I arrived at my hotel and the time I was to meet a client for dinner. I quickly changed clothes and ran the stairwells of my hotel. You can also carry a jump rope (an excellent exercise tool) in your luggage. I have found that exercise enables me to function better during a stressful day on the road. It relaxes me, reduces stress, and seems to improve mental processing.

3. *"I am so busy from the time I get up to the time I go to bed that I am just too tired to exercise."* Let's face it; sometimes we *are* too tired to exercise. If, however, you find yourself tired all the time, something needs to change in your life. Perhaps you need more sleep. Maybe you need to reprioritize your time.

As we get older and our bodies begin to wear down, exercise can actually energize us, enabling us to accomplish more. Of course, there are going to be days when physical activity is drudgery. However, more often than not, if you push through the fatigue, you will find your tiredness begins to dissipate. Exercise can help you sleep better and stimulate mental activities. Short-term tiredness is not an automatic cue that you should curtail exercise. Just the opposite may be true. By eating right and exercising regularly, you will find more energy to do the things that are most important in your life.

Vickie Farris is a forty-something, home-schooling mother of ten. She says one of her only solutions for emotional, physical, and spiritual restoration is her daily walk. "I fight for that four-mile walk every day. This is basically the only free time I have, but it is all I really need to keep going. 'Mom's walk' is one of the permanent items in my daily plan."[1]

4. *"When the weather is bad, I can't get motivated to do much of anything."* It's too hot in New Orleans, Dallas, Atlanta, or Miami in the summer. I have been in each of these cities during the summer months, and running outside is next to impossible. I have also been in Minneapolis in the snow, Seattle in the rain, and Phoenix in the heat. Let's face it; no matter where we live or travel, the weather is not going to be perfect for outdoor activities *all* the time. Learn to adapt your activities to your particular climate. Exercise indoors when you must. Enjoy seasonal sports or activities when you can. Hot weather exercise requires proper hydration. Cold weather exercise requires adequate clothing or equipment. During bad weather months, always have a contingency plan. If you can't exercise outdoors, think about what you can do as an alternative. In some cities, there are groups that walk inside local malls during the winter months. This provides both a physical and social outlet.

5. *"I would exercise if I had the right equipment."* You don't need expensive, gym-quality exercise equipment to stay in shape. As I mentioned earlier, a jump rope is an inexpensive and very effective piece of equipment. A good pair of shoes for walking and a wind or rain suit during spring or fall is adequate. Those of us forced indoors during certain months of the year can still get a good aerobic workout by riding a stationary bicycle or using a jogging or

walking machine. If you can afford it, join a health club or gym where you can get instruction and enjoy the camaraderie of working out with others.

When Is the Right Time to Exercise?

The truth is, there is no right time. Each of us has a different schedule and varying preferences. The majority of us exercise early in the morning, before the day gets too busy, or at the end of the day, after our busy day is nearly over. When I used to commute to work in Los Angeles, life was stressful. Exercise at the end of the day was a way to reduce my stress, and I looked forward to it. My preference has always been to work out in the afternoon. By the end of the day, my muscles are warmed up and ready to go.

There are many people who prefer to start their day with exercise. If something unexpected comes along later in the day, they don't have to worry about abandoning their workout. If you choose to exercise early in the day, be sure to stretch adequately beforehand; there is greater risk of injury when the muscles are cold. Still others try to work out on their lunch break. After daylight-saving time kicks into effect in the fall, it is dark by the time I leave work, so occasionally I will adjust my schedule to get in a run during my lunch hour.

If you travel, the time you work out will likely have to be flexible with your schedule. People who follow tight routines find it difficult to adjust. I know I do. Still, the bottom line is to get your exercise in *whenever* you can. There is rarely the need to forgo a workout just because you are on the road. Schedule time for a run, long walk, or a workout at the hotel gym. If your stay involves an overnight at someone's home, tell your host ahead of time that you need a half-hour or an hour to exercise. Encourage them to join you, if they can.

"Now I Lay Me Down to Sleep"

In our fast-paced world, it is easy to forget another important element to overall health—adequate sleep. Most of us get less sleep than we really need. Does this come as a surprise? We cannot deprive ourselves of adequate sleep to compensate for a busy lifestyle. In addition, sleep efficiency—the proportion of time you actually spend asleep when you're in bed—declines steadily throughout life. From a peak of 95 percent in your twenties, it slides to about 75 percent by age seventy. The good news is that regular exercise can help. Research shows that regular exercise improves the quality of sleep and decreases the amount of time it takes to fall asleep.[2] As we work toward increasing activity during the day, some of us need to work toward getting a good night's sleep.

Studies indicate that lack of sleep interferes with our immune system, raises our blood pressure, and leads to general fatigue and unproductiveness (reducing mental work by as much as 25 percent). Americans sleep 20 percent less than our ancestors did a century ago. The National Commission on Sleep Disorders estimates 60 million of us are chronically sleep deprived.[3] What are the positive results of getting enough sleep? Sleep helps to lower blood pressure, increase feelings of happiness, build and repair the body's cells, and improve immune defenses—to name just a few.

The sleep we do get needs to be a restful sleep. Merely laying our heads down does not turn off our brains. Some of us lie there frantically reviewing our day, thinking of all that needs to be done tomorrow. When we finally drop off to sleep, we often find it is

Dr. Gregory Jantz on Merging Body and Spirit

All of us can identify with what has been called "the tyranny of the urgent." The urgent matters in our lives seem to overtake even those things we consider important. Like a pinball, we are constantly whacked from one place to another by the paddles of the urgent. In the midst of this frantic activity, many people conclude they simply don't have the time for fitness.

In his book *Too Busy Not to Pray,* Bill Hybels, pastor of Willow Creek Church, suggests that the busier people are, the more time they need to devote to prayer. In other words, the more things they have going on in their day, the more they need the power and strength that prayer can provide. Why? Because only with the help and strength of God and His Spirit can you possibly do everything you need to do!

Prayer provides spiritual strength and energy. The spiritual and physical work together. This is the way God created us. In 1 Corinthians 9:24-27, our spiritual life in Christ is likened by the apostle Paul to a physical race. Our spiritual efforts for the kingdom are likened to the various parts of the physical body. The discipline gained through physical activity is used by Paul as a lesson for spiritual stamina.

In the midst of a busy day, you can combine the two. You can use the time of physical activity as a time of spiritual meditation or prayer. How about listening to the Bible on tape or to Christian music while walking or jogging? Both prayer and aerobic exercise have been shown to produce feelings of well-being and to relieve stress.

restless, not restorative. If this describes you, try this: As you lie down, take some time to thank God for each night that He gives you rest. Meditate on verses like Psalm 16:9, "Therefore my heart is glad and my tongue rejoices; my body also will rest secure." Let the anxieties of the day go (don't dwell on them), and refuse to think about the perceived troubles of tomorrow. Your mind may want to race, but follow your breathing and rest with a spirit of thankfulness. Or consider listening to instrumental music that produces relaxation and calm at the end of a busy day.

What does sleep have to do with exercise as we get older? Exercise is effort. Effort is best performed when you are rested to begin with. Sometimes the best thing you can do during your busy day is to make sure you get a good and restful sleep the night before.

Avoid the Easy Path

Escalators, people movers, elevators—these are all designed to make our lives easier. And sometimes we need them. Most often, however, we use them simply because they are there. Let's look at some of the choices you can make in your everyday life to build strength or stamina by making slight adjustments in your daily habits.

- Park your car at the far end of the parking lot and walk. (You will get fewer dings on your car door too!)
- Walk up stairs rather than take elevators.
- Avoid escalators, elevators, or people-movers in airports or malls.
- Take your dirty clothes to the laundry room instead of throwing them in the hamper.

- Walk upstairs for that glass of water instead of yelling at your kids to bring it to you.
- Walk around the block on your lunch break.
- Take a walk with your dog, spouse, kids, or a friend after dinner instead of sitting in front of the television.

While these may not seem like much individually, taken together, day after day and week after week, they increase the amount of time your body is moving, burning calories, and strengthening muscles. By making a conscious effort to counteract our sedentary lifestyles, we can reap enormous long-term benefits such as longer and more productive lives.

Tom Mason on Finding Time for Fitness

The common complaint among overweight and apparently unfit people I meet is that there is not enough time for working out and staying fit. On the other hand, there are undeniably busy and high-achieving people who *do* find time to invest in their physical health. So what is the difference between these two kinds of people?

There is no resource in life that has been handed out as equally as the resource of time. We each have differing amounts of money, looks, and intelligence. But we all have the exact same amount of time in a day. So it is not that people who stay fit have more of this precious commodity. They just use it better. They are better organized and consider fitness a higher priority than the unfit group.

In my own case, the commitment to maintaining a regular fitness schedule has been interrupted on occasion by illness, injury, or other obstacles. Yet I have been motivated to get fit and stay fit for over twenty years. During this time I have had significant corporate positions requiring extensive travel and schedules that last well into the evening hours. What I have found is that most days are unpredictable as to the late afternoon and evening hours and that even if time is available at the end of the day, my energy level has waned to the point I can seldom generate enough enthusiasm to work out.

On the front end of the day, however, there is almost always an open opportunity to exercise. The early morning can provide as much time as anyone needs for a fitness program. If more time is needed, simply get up earlier. There is virtually an unlimited horizon before the start of the day. It is no surprise, then, that morning exercisers are the most consistent over time.

But what about the extra hour of sleep? Again, it is a matter of priority, and it is establishing priority that separates the fit from the unfit. The person who truly values working out will make it a related priority to retire earlier for the night since he or she must rise early to begin the day with a workout. All priorities end up working together.

My own exercise of choice is running. It can be done virtually anywhere. It requires only simple clothing, which is easily packed. And to be outdoors running in the quiet of the early morning is peaceful and intoxicating. In short, laziness may be a valid excuse for not exercising, but not having enough time is not. Equally valid is simply admitting that physical fitness is not as high a priority as other activities that fill your day, from reading to watching television, from taking a nap to attending a party. Regular exercise will never become a way of life until fitness becomes a high priority so as to force its way into the day's activities.

Fitness Time Management

Tom Mason is right. Time is a precious resource. There will always be demands for us to do something other than what we have planned. So I encourage you to schedule your workout into each week. Decide ahead of time what will constitute a true crisis and what will merely be something to sidetrack you from your routine. You decide; don't let others decide for you. While this might sound inflexible, there are very few things I allow to get in the way of a daily workout. This is not to say I am not willing to adjust my time to fit in an important meeting or a special event, but I find a way. The way we use our time every day determines our priorities in life.

If you are getting started, let your loved ones know how important your new routine is to you. Once you set your priorities, stick with them. Treat the magnificent machine God has given you with care and find the time to do proper maintenance. To the extent that you honor the temple God has given you, it will serve you with greater efficiency.

Now let's take a brief look at several busy people who have discovered the value of making exercise a priority in their lives.

Nani is a forty-year-old single mom and an administrator for a nursing home. In high school she was active, but when she got married, had children, and started working, she began adding unwanted pounds. She remained inactive for nearly twenty years before coming to the realization that she was overweight and out of shape. Nani wisely didn't try to solve all her problems overnight. Instead, she started slowly. She began a class in water aerobics and then graduated to floor aerobics. Today she combines running and walking on a treadmill, uses a rowing machine and exercycle, and does strength training. Her favorite time to work out is in the morning, giving her more time to spend with her children later in the day. For women trying to get started with an exercise program, she offers this advice: "Make exercise a priority and do something every day."

George is an eighty-three-year-old former corporate executive and leader of a Christian ministry. Although he has slowed down a bit since his forties, he has a sharp mind and trim body. He always carries his luggage through airports and continues to walk thirty minutes a day, five days a week. Occasionally he rides an exercycle. At fifty-nine, George started going to a gym, and he has remained active ever since. His advice for seniors is to "Get up and get going. Do what you can. Don't make it too hard or you will be tempted to quit."

Michael is a fifty-two-year-old accountant and master swimmer (someone who competes in swim meets specially designed for those over forty). He has missed just six pool workouts in the past five months. Although his office is busiest during tax season, he still manages to schedule a two-hour lunch so he can get his workout in. He encourages people to make the space for exercise and then cherish that space. "Most people don't make the time in the day," he says. His advice: "The key is to set aside specific time and begin to set up a regular structure—even if it is only fifteen minutes a day."

Putting Our Lives in Perspective

There are events and seasons in our lives that we can look back on now and think, "Why did I waste so much of my time fretting over that?" Or we can look at activities that have robbed us of precious time that could have been used in more productive ways. Sometimes these time-robbing activities are subtle—like television.

(By the time the average American reaches sixty-five, she will have spent nine years watching TV!) As we give an inventory of our lives before our Maker, just how will we justify some of the unwise ways we have spent our time here on earth?

Because many of us are up against seemingly urgent matters, we often lose sight of what is really important. In his book *Trusting God Through Tears,* Jehu Burton tells the story of losing his teenage son to a brain aneurysm. When he finally returned to his engineering job, he saw the petty squabbles between coworkers and arguments in staff meetings from a different perspective. In light of losing his son, these things seemed insignificant. What so many of us lack in today's fast-paced world is exactly what Burton found: perspective. Often God gets our attention through a crisis, injury, or unexpected event. During these tough times, we need one another, and we need an eternal perspective about the things that matter most in life. And one of the ways to determine what matters most is to ask ourselves whether the activities we choose will matter twenty or thirty years from now. Will they matter in eternity?

During his acceptance speech to the Road Racing Hall of Fame, Alberto Salazar offered his own life perspective. "Whatever we accomplish in life, if it's solely for our own good, then it doesn't mean that much. The things you do that affect others in a positive way are the ones that count. Whatever facet of life you are in, God has given you a gift; do the best you can with that gift."[4]

Evalyn, an eighty-two-year-old widow, puts her motivation for staying healthy in eternal terms. "There is only one reason I continue to exercise: to help other people. I wake up every day and say, 'Thank you, Lord. Here I am again.'" Exercise may profit little, as the apostle Paul explained, but for people like Evalyn, eating healthy and staying active is a means to helping others. "All one needs to do is to look around and see the need. I'm just glad I am still able to do something about it."

So now you're ready to make the time. How can you motivate yourself to make the most of it? Where does motivation to stay healthy come from? How do we maintain it once we have finally mastered it? It all starts with having a plan.

Motivation: Finding and Keeping Momentum

DON OTIS

I try not to get too caught up thinking about the task ahead.
I just do what has to be done. I have the belief in myself
that what I'm doing is right. Then I let the rest happen.

—EAMONN COGHLAN, THE ONLY RUNNER OVER FORTY

TO BREAK THE FOUR-MINUTE MILE

The pattern is the same every year. People make resolutions, and by the first week of January I can anticipate more new faces at the gym. Yet like everything else that we think we ought to be doing, once the drudgery starts getting to us, we give up our goals for dieting and exercise. By late spring the crowds have dwindled, and the fitness equipment is available again until the next cycle hits the following January.

It doesn't have to be like that. If you are one of the people who has started a routine at some point and then given up, don't be discouraged. If you have tried to maintain an exercise routine or diet in the past and failed, I want to provide some practical ideas to keep you focused. That's what this chapter is about: keeping you moving forward in healthy activity for as long as you live.

Have you ever wondered why some people are just more goal oriented and focused than others? They can set their minds to something and stick with it under the most adverse circumstances. For most of us, finding motivation is a major challenge. As we get older, it becomes even more difficult to establish new patterns in our lives. As we age, we become more set in comfortable routines. These patterns are difficult to change. Just recognizing this fact in your own life may be the starting point for developing healthy new habits.

Pam is a forty-nine-year-old mother and grandmother who works full time at a local utility company. She started to attend Weight Watchers meetings a dozen years ago. Soon she added exercise to her new lifestyle because she wanted to lose more weight. As Pam began to shed pounds, she felt better and began to look better. Today she says she just doesn't feel right if she is not consistently active. If she gets tired of her exercise routine, Pam simply changes it and does something else for a few weeks. Her primary emphasis is on aerobic exercise—jogging, walking, cycling, and using a stair machine. She also lifts weights to stay toned. Pam is a perfect example of someone who was not physically active until just before she turned forty.

Why are some people naturally motivated, while others don't seem to care? What does it take to motivate ourselves or others? Is there a key to motivating ourselves to do what we already know is good for us? I wish I could say I have perfect answers for everyone. I don't. Each of us is motivated by something entirely different. Some of us are motivated by how we look, others by fear, still others tend to be more goal directed. What tends to motivate you? Whatever it is, the key is to find a way to transfer good habits and discipline from one area of your life to a new one.

John is a sixty-one-year-old recovered alcoholic. He is in better shape today than he was twenty years ago. What motivates him to get up early each day for exercise? He says the rewards of exercise are that he feels better, has more energy, is mentally sharper, and experiences less stress. John can also do physical activities he wouldn't otherwise be able to do. Perhaps the most important benefit he derives from physical exercise is that his discipline spills over into his prayer life. Of course, there are days when exercise feels like work. During these times, he takes a few days off and comes back fresh later.

It is no secret that as we get older it gets harder to learn a new language or important skill, such as how to use emerging technology. It comes as no surprise that your children or grandchildren are often better equipped (in most instances) to program a remote control or find information quickly on the Internet. We didn't grow up with these technologies, so our tendency is to shy away from them. *We avoid the things that we don't feel comfortable with.* This is a natural human reaction. Now translate this discomfort into a new sport, activity, or trip to the gym.

As I've gotten older, I have discovered a few things about exercise. First, it is easier to get out of shape than it is to get in shape. Another thing I have reluctantly accepted (well, almost) is that my body does not feel the same as it did when I was in my late twenties. I try to tell this to people who are in their twenties, and they give me blank stares. And why shouldn't they? They can't relate to what you and I are discovering. Muscle elasticity is not what it once was. We feel increased soreness after vigorous exercise. We don't have the leg speed or agility we once did. And recovery time increases with the intensity of our exercise. As someone who has always been active, it may be easier for me to see the differences between my teens, twenties, thirties, and forties. If you have been less active and are just getting started, you may have no point of reference. People who were active in their teens and twenties cannot assume they can pick up where they left off. The so-called weekend warriors—those who engage in high intensity, competitive activities—often find themselves succumbing to a medley of injuries, mostly due to overuse or improper stretching.

Anytime you start something new, you can expect to feel some degree of discomfort. Minor aches and pains are a normal consequence of increased activity. More important, however, is how you will feel mentally when venturing into the unknown. Whenever we do anything new, we experience some degree of anxiety or even embarrassment. These feelings will dissipate as you forge ahead and the activities become easier. If it is an activity that requires some level of skill, get the help or instruction you need in the beginning. Or better yet, join others who can give you the advice and encouragement you need to get started.

If you are forty, fifty, or sixty and have never stepped into a gym, it can be an intimidating experience. It is a bit like sitting in the cockpit of a 747 for the first time. You look at all the lights, levers, and buttons and wonder how anyone can remember what they are all for. In a health club, everyone seems to know how to use the equipment, but to a newcomer it can look as complicated and daunting as that jet cockpit. What's more, everyone there may seem to be in better shape than you. You might secretly think, "This is not for me," or "This is for people who are already in really good shape." Neither of these assessments would be true. Are gyms only for people who are in great shape? Of course not. Most of us have been in not-so-good shape at some point in our lives (or may be there now!). How do we get in better shape if we avoid the very places that will help us to improve?

Good Reasons to Get Motivated Now

Following are a few good reasons for starting or keeping an active fitness regimen. You may already know most of these by heart, but it helps to reinforce them.

1. *Exercise is physically good for you.* People who exercise regularly reduce the risk of heart disease, diabetes, and high blood pressure. Exercise also helps control cholesterol.

2. *Exercise will help you live longer.* Even those who are moderately active on a regular basis have lower mortality rates than those who are inactive.

3. *Exercise is good for your mental health.* Studies show that taking invigorating walks or engaging in other forms of exercise give older people's brains a good workout, increasing memory and sharpening judgment.[1]

4. *Exercise helps reduce stress.* Physical activity is a natural way to manage or release stress in our lives. Regular aerobic exercise does more than just lessen the fight-or-flight feeling. It improves the

body's ability to handle the effects of stress by keeping immunity high and protecting cells from damage.

5. *Exercise helps relieve depression.* Regular exercise lifts depression just as well as prescription anti-depressants.[2]

6. *Exercise facilitates weight loss and weight control.* People who exercise burn more calories, which aids in weight reduction.

7. *Exercise can improve your physical appearance.* Those who engage in regular physical activities are generally leaner and have better muscle definition.

8. *Exercise stimulates fat-clearing enzymes.* Exercise speeds the breakdown of fat.[3]

9. *Exercise plays a pivotal role in sexuality.* Exercise enhances libido by increasing blood flow.

10. *Exercise enables us to be more productive and capable of carrying on God's work.* People who are healthy and fit can accomplish more for the kingdom of God.

No Easy Solution

Who can forget Nike's slogan "Just Do It"? For those of us who have always "just done it," we need little prompting. The reason? It has become a habit—the activity has become a part of our lives. Nevertheless, most people are not motivated by three-word slogans. Instead, the pressure to "just do it" can create feelings of guilt or of falling short of what they should be doing. Nor are we necessarily motivated by seeing a well-conditioned athlete wincing through the last few grueling miles of a marathon. Realistically, this discourages more of us than it inspires. Motivation comes from within each of us. People who achieve small goals or accomplish great things do so because they are able to make small sacrifices. The same is true for you. Getting started, establishing a plan, reaching our goals—each of these is about overcoming mental obstacles first. As we will see later in this chapter, there are some practical ways you can make your journey easier.

There is one rule that has helped me to stay focused and active during more than thirty years of regular exercise: *Consistency is more important than intensity.* We have all seen friends or family start and stop exercising or dieting to lose weight over and over again. Why do they do this? It is because they assume their diet or exercise is a temporary solution to a long-term problem. If it takes twenty years to get out of shape or become overweight, what makes us think we can get in shape in a couple of weeks? It won't happen. Generally speaking, it takes about twenty-one days of practice for anything to become a new habit. And even after we make it through those first twenty-one days, exercise will not suddenly get easier. It will, however, be easier to overcome the day-to-day mental obstacles that used to be excuses for not doing it.

There are days I don't feel like doing anything. You will feel this way too. Expect it. The good news is that on about 50 percent of these doldrums days I find my mind has been playing tricks on me. After I get started, the malaise disappears. The other half of the time I just go through the motions, feeling undermotivated through my entire workout. If you feel like this, revise your expectations. Slow down and reduce your normal intensity. If you wait to feel good before exercising, chances are you won't do it. That isn't to say you should feel guilty if you take off a day or two; sometimes a break from a regular routine is exactly what we need to stay motivated over the long haul. Rest can rejuvenate us and provide energy and enthusiasm for our next workout.

Keys to Getting Started and Staying Motivated

At the risk of alienating my brother George, I want to share a personal story of how I got started running. George is two and a half years older than I am. The age difference doesn't mean much now, but it sure did when I was a kid! My motivation to run goes all the way back to my childhood. Running meant survival. It began when I would bolt out of the house and down the street to escape my irate brother, who was pretty fast himself! There was another way I learned to elude the viselike headlocks he administered. George was afraid of heights, so I would climb onto the roof of our Los Angeles home when I got tired of running.

Running and climbing became the only two ways I could escape impending danger from my older sibling. They also kept me active. Thankfully, today I don't need an older brother to keep me motivated. If you are one of the millions of people who didn't have an older brother as I did, here are some practical steps to help you get started or keep going.

Start Slow and Keep Going

Without exception, the dozens of over-forty people whom I have interviewed for this book tell me the key to getting started is to do whatever you can—even if it is a small amount. It is always better to start small and slow with a new diet or exercise routine. Our tendency is to try to do too much too soon, because we want to see results.

People who start too fast, however, are not prepared in body or mind. Remember this principle: *It is better to start slow and stay in the race than to start fast and have to quit later.* Starting too fast is a sure way to become discouraged. You will lose any enjoyment you receive from your sport or exercise program. Be patient. The results will come from your commitment to a consistent schedule.

View your exercise routine as a permanent lifestyle change, not a temporary fix. Allow it to become as much a part of your life as anything else. While exercise should not take precedence over family, church, or marriage, it must begin to assume a higher priority in your life. Otherwise anything and everything can become more important and, before you know it, you become discouraged because you have missed a week of workouts. Minor crises have a way of changing our routines and upending our plans. Unless the crisis is real, don't let these distractions deter you from taking care of yourself.

Pacing is important. I like to run on a track several months out of the year because it trains my body to feel what it is like to run at a particular speed. Once I get out on the open road, I have a fairly good idea whether I am running at a six-and-a half- or seven-and-a-half-minute mile. Our spiritual lives follow similar patterns. I have known people who became Christians and are like the seed that was sown on rocky soil in Jesus' parable of the sower. They spring up and are scorched by the sun. They burn out. Nearly every aspect of our lives is about pacing ourselves effectively. Good athletes understand this. As we get older, pacing is simply a matter of wisdom.

There is another reason for starting slow: the potential for injuries. Your body needs time to adapt to the new physical stress you are putting on it. Even if you are in excellent shape, you need to ease into new sports and new activities. Our bodies and various muscle groups become accustomed to certain regular movements. When we introduce a new activity or sport, it increases the chance of injury until our muscles can make the necessary adjustments. The same is true for seasonal activities like hiking or skiing. Before hitting the trails or the slopes, make sure you work the specific muscle groups used in these activities.

KEEP A JOURNAL

I have a stack of four-by-six-inch cards in my desk. These help me keep track of my activities and running. Each day I mark the distance, route, time, and any unusual conditions, like weather. At the gym I have another card for weight training that includes weight amounts and repetitions. I always know how a particular workout compares with other days. No one cares but me, yet it provides a measure of self-accountability. It also offers me the data I need to chart my progress, consistency, or times from month to month or year to year. Those who keep a log of their daily or weekly exercise are more likely to maintain their fitness routine.

You can make your journal as simple or as elaborate as you want. Use it to hold yourself accountable if you exercise alone (which I do). It also can help you make adjustments in your workout or exercise routine; if you find yourself getting stale, bored, or unmotivated, don't be afraid to make changes in your workout.

Set Goals

Someone once said, "If you don't know where you are going, any road will take you there." What do you want to accomplish with your exercise routine? Of course we all want to be healthy and look our best. These goals, however, are too general. Get specific. Set short- and long-term goals, and track your progress along the way.

Let me give you a personal example. My goals are ongoing. In other words, each year for the past twenty years one of my goals has been to run one thousand miles a year. To achieve this, I have to be consistent and average just over eighty-three miles each month. By keeping track of my progress, I know exactly how close I am to achieving my goal. I also have smaller goals, such as running certain times or entering specific races. These are goals that I can reach throughout the year, even as I work toward my bigger goal.

Your own goals should be challenging but also realistic (more on this later). Don't be discouraged, however, if you set a goal and can't achieve it at first. Keep working at it.

Eliminate Boredom

I hear people say how boring it is to swim or run. "I could never do that," they exclaim. For me, there are countless ways to break up the monotony of swimming or running or anything else. In swimming, there are different strokes, interval training, or change of location. In running, you can do hills, trails, parks, tracks, or indoor machines. You can go fast or slow, up or down, in groups or on your own.

You can also reduce boredom through cross-training (see chapter 7), goal setting, or changing environments. If you like to walk the exact same route every day at exactly the same time of day, that's great! Personally, I like variety. I like new challenges. If you find yourself losing interest, a change of scenery may be just the thing to relieve the tedium.

One important note: In gyms as well as outdoors, it has become common to see people exercising while listening to radios or CD players. While this can make the time seem to go by faster, it can be downright dangerous. If you walk, run, or ride outdoors, headphones limit your ability to avoid danger. Limit your use of these devices to those times when you're exercising in a controlled environment, such as indoors.

Find a Friend

An exercise companion can break the monotony while offering accountability. Most of us don't like to work out alone. If you find it difficult to get started on your own, find someone who will do it with you. Or get involved in a group activity such as walking, aerobics, or spinning (stationary cycling). In addition to motivation, there are other advantages to having a partner. If you are a woman who enjoys walking, hiking, jogging, or biking outside, it is safer to do it with a partner. In addition, a partner can help encourage you to improve.

Try to find someone who is at the same fitness level before agreeing to a regular routine. If you are competitive and want to improve, you need someone who will push you as much as you will push them. Just as a good partner can help you to improve your level of fitness, a weak partner can do just the opposite. Discuss your individual goals and fitness levels before making a commitment. And don't be afraid to change partners if you find that you are incompatible—having schedules, goals, or personalities that are not in sync.

Set a Specific Time

As we briefly mentioned in the first chapter, there is no best time to exercise. The challenge is to fit it in when it is most convenient for you. Keena, a forty-two-year-old mother of four boys, says it takes a conscious choice to make time for the activities she enjoys. She finds time in her busy day to get in a game or two of tennis, racquetball, squash, or a kick-boxing class.

The key is to schedule time for your activities and protect that time. Just as you wouldn't interrupt your quiet time spent reading the Bible or in prayer, guard the time you set apart for your fitness activities. Setting a specific time for exercise makes it easier to develop the exercise habit.

Learn a New Sport

Are you one of those people who, like me, gets used to doing things the same way year after year? I was forty before I finally took my first downhill skiing lessons. The instructor who taught me couldn't get me to stop on my own. Finally he skied backward in front of me to provide more braking power. It took awhile, but I finally learned to snowplow. Now I can enjoy skiing with my two snowboarding sons. At forty-one, I learned to water ski when a friend nearly threw me off his boat for a lesson. At forty-two, I learned to play golf, thanks to the prodding of my oldest son, Justin. At forty-three, I learned how to play squash as an alternate activity during the winter months.

Not all activities interest me, nor do I always enjoy everything new that I try. Yet I've found that an alternative sport or activity can be fun and provide motivation to stay active. Don't be afraid to try something new—even if, as in my case, you are embarrassed in the process!

HAVE FUN

I know what you're thinking. "Does he really mean *fun?*" If you absolutely hate doing something, chances are you will find a reason—any reason—to stop doing it. So the obvious solution is to find an activity that you enjoy. Benji Durden, a former Olympic marathoner, offers the following advice: "If you want to stay motivated, running [or any other activity] has to be more than something you do mechanically. It has to be fun. And if it's not, it's probably time to shift to a whole new view, to examine what you are doing and change it."[4]

REGULARLY DO SOMETHING DIFFERENT

We have already talked about the value of learning a new sport or activity. Cross-training also offers a welcome change. Cross-training is simply substituting a variety of exercises or activities for what you normally do. For example, instead of walking or running, you might break up your week by including a bike ride, a swim, a game of tennis, or a hike.

ACCEPT YOUR LIMITATIONS

At twenty or thirty you might have been able to do things you can't do today. Don't get depressed. Instead, adjust to it. Most races today include age-group categories. See how you stack up against other people *your age.* Change your goals to reflect reality.

Ken is fifty-seven and each year ranks in the top five runners within his age group at the annual Lilac Bloomsday Road Race in Spokane, Washington. He has finished in the top one hundred out of fifty thousand runners! He is fast, running a mile in well under six minutes. But he is also smart about his running. When he reaches the point in his training where his knees start hurting, he cycles, swims, and does stationary running in the pool to lessen the impact on his body. Though Ken knows when he is pushing his knees too hard, eventually he will have to change sports or lessen the intensity of his running. By revising your goals and participating in different activities, you can reduce the possibility of injury.

INVOLVE YOUR CHILDREN

If you have children at home, include them in your activities. Riding, basketball, hiking, canoeing, and cross-country skiing are all fun things you can enjoy as a family. My brother and I have six boys between us. When we get together, we find a gym or basketball court and play some pretty intense games. Last summer we climbed the twelve-thousand-foot Mount Adams!

Whether you walk through a park, hike the trail to a waterfall, or play a court sport, consider involving your children or grandchildren with you. Even if they say they don't want to at first, they are usually glad later on. Some of the best talks I have had with my sons have been while we were splitting firewood together, riding bicycles, or lifting weights. Christian parents can use physical activities as a means of communicating values and further developing relationships with their children.

Staying Motivated on the Road

In today's fast-paced world, people are on the go more than ever before. For people who travel frequently, making regular time for exercise poses a special problem. Among other things, they are dealing with time zone changes, long workdays, diverse (or nonexistent) equipment, and variable outdoor conditions. If you are a frequent traveler, you can't afford *not* to work out while you are on the road.

Many hotels now have adequate fitness facilities. During a convention in Orlando, I trained for a ten-kilometer race on the indoor running machine at my hotel. When I used to fly from Los Angeles to Tel Aviv for business, the first thing I did after finding my hotel room was to jog three or four miles along the Mediterranean shoreline. After sitting for seventeen hours, it felt good to stretch my legs and get some fresh air.

In the next few years we will begin to see airport exercise clubs, places where busy travelers can grab a workout between flights.

It isn't always easy to fit exercise into a busy travel schedule. But you *can* find ways to do it. Whether you pack a jump rope, walk around the parking lot of your hotel, climb the stairs, or use a hotel's fitness facilities, you don't have to sacrifice your workout while you are on the road.

THREE

Getting Started After Forty

MARYANNA YOUNG

The simplest way to preserve health is to exercise. It is the only lifestyle change that does not raise additional questions: Exercise equals health, period.

—DR. GEORGE SHEEHAN

You will never see a photo of fifty-two-year-old Kris on a Wheaties box. Nor are you likely to find her entering a local road race or swim meet. Her daughters are now in college, and she is busy teaching third graders. In their free time, Kris and her husband enjoy outdoor activities like boating, hiking, and skiing. Yet she has never cared much for organized sports or exercise classes. In fact, she is starting to find normal activities—like gardening or hiking—to be increasingly difficult. Sometimes she feels tired and out of breath. Though she is careful about what she eats, lately she has found it tough to keep her weight stable.

   Kris and countless others like her realize they need to do something to combat the inevitable effects of time. The question is, "Where do they begin?" This chapter is for those who have started an exercise routine and found themselves unable or unwilling to continue. It is also for those who, like Kris, have *never* exercised. And it is for those who have started and quit exercise programs so many times they feel embarrassed and frustrated.

Finding a Personal Purpose

While no amount of exercise can absolutely guarantee long life, exercise can improve the chances that you will live a healthier life. Along with a positive attitude and healthy diet, your level of fitness plays an enormous role in how well you feel, what illnesses you avoid, and how much you enjoy life. No matter how old you are, it is never too late to get started. No matter what shape you are in, you can dramatically improve the state of your health. The hardest part of getting started is taking those first three steps out the door.

One of the keys is to commit to make exercise a part of your daily routine. Like any other good habit, the goal is to make it part of your lifestyle, and that will happen only when you incorporate exercise into your day-to-day activities.

To make exercise part of your life, you need a *personal purpose* for starting or continuing to work out. This can be anything from losing weight, prolonging your years, improving your figure, or staving off disease. Additional positive benefits to staying active include:

- It improves and strengthens the cardiovascular system (by improving the oxygen supply to all parts of the body, including the heart, muscles, and the brain).
- It increases the level of muscle strength and muscle endurance.

- It increases the body's basal metabolic rate, which helps you burn calories even when resting.
- It improves your body's ability to use fat for energy during physical activity.
- It helps to maintain weight loss with better results than dieting alone.
- It increases your maximal oxygen uptake (the best measure of your physical working capacity).
- It gives you more energy to meet the demands of everyday life and provides a reserve to respond to unexpected emergencies.
- It helps alleviate lower back pain and decreases the likelihood of lower back problems.
- It improves the function of your immune system, enabling you to fight off sickness or disease.
- It assists in reducing anxiety and decreases the chance of developing tension headaches.
- It helps preserve lean body tissue.
- It can reduce medical and healthcare expenses as you get older.
- It reduces the risk of developing high blood pressure.
- It improves both the quantity and quality of your sleep.
- It lowers your heart rate (we will discuss this benefit in a moment) and makes your heart pump more efficiently.
- It improves your overall quality of life (by enabling you to do activities you could not otherwise do) and improves mental alertness.
- It helps regulate blood glucose levels, which can help to prevent the onset of diabetes.

There are many reasons to begin or maintain an exercise program. Which one will be your own personal purpose? While we can
examine all the good reasons to stay active, the fact remains that each
of us must come to grips with the very personal decision to keep at
it. By creating a "personal reasons" list, you can occasionally remind
yourself why you got started in the first place. On those days when
working out might be the *last* thing you want to do, reviewing your
own personal list may be all the boost you need to get up and get
going. For example:

> "I want more energy so I can enjoy doing the things
> I have always done."

> "I want more energy to spend quality time with
> family or friends."

> "I want to be able to climb stairs or do activities
> without becoming breathless."

> "I want to set my children or grandchildren an
> example of enjoyment of outdoor activities."

> "I want to have the stamina to help others or
> minister more effectively."

I was always involved in sports as a child and into college.
After I graduated, I didn't take exercise as seriously. I remember the
catalyst that turned me around and gave me a personal purpose
for continuing. I was on a vacation in the rugged Sawtooth
Mountains of central Idaho. At the time, my exercise routine was
inconsistent at best—especially when compared with my years
in competitive sports. Although I was fit enough to complete
the day hike with friends, I was shocked by my elevated heart

rate and shortness of breath. It was that single experience that caused me to reevaluate my need to make exercise a regular part of my life again.

Now let's look at how increasing your level of activity can have a long-term positive impact on your health. The good news is that if you are new to exercise, even small amounts of regular, sustained activity can help you live longer and healthier.

KEEPING FIT LOWERS YOUR HEART RATE

The truth is, your heart never fully rests. It pumps millions of gallons of blood throughout your lifetime. The only time your heart gets a break is during the two-thirds of a second between heartbeats! When you begin an exercise routine, though, the increase in physical activity actually lowers your resting heart rate. This in turn allows your heart more rest between beats.

Here is the formula you need to use to be sure you are getting an adequate aerobic workout for your age. Simply subtract your age from 220 to determine your maximum heart rate. For instance, if you are 50 years old, your maximum heart rate is 170. Your personal goal is to work up to 70 percent of your capacity—in this case, about 120 beats per minute.

The average resting heart rate for American men is seventy-two beats per minutes; for women, it is about eighty beats per minute. By reducing your resting heart rate just ten beats per minute through regular exercise, here's how much less work your heart would have to do:

- 10 fewer beats per minute means a savings of 600 beats in one hour
- 600 fewer beats per hour means a savings of 14,400 beats every day

- 14,400 fewer beats each day equals a total savings of 5,256,000 beats per year

Imagine: By lowering your heart rate just ten beats per minute, you are giving your heart an additional month of rest over the course of a year!

Not As Hard As You Might Think

Dr. Kenneth Cooper is known as the father of aerobics because he is the one who started us all thinking about the long-term benefits of sustaining activity. He is now seventy years old and continues his work through his world-renowned clinic in Dallas, Texas. He recommends that before starting an exercise program, there are four key steps to take:

1. Start with a thorough physical evaluation.
2. Approach exercise as an educational process.
3. Embrace lifestyle changes that are safe, effective, and realistic.
4. Commit to a process for reevaluation.[1]

If you start as Cooper suggests, the next steps are not nearly as difficult as you might think. How many times have you heard the phrase "No pain, no gain"? We don't have to torture ourselves to enjoy the benefits of exercise. In America we have swallowed the idea that if a little of anything is good, a lot is better. This doesn't always hold true with exercise—especially as we get older. Nor does our activity have to be overly intense to still be of value. Unfortunately, far too many people begin an exercise program that is too difficult, and they get burned out too quickly. So if this has happened to you in the past, keep the following three rules in mind.

- Keep it simple. Just make sure the time you spend working out includes aerobic exercise as the cornerstone of your program.
- Keep it fun. If it isn't fun, you won't keep doing it.
- Keep at it. Measure your success with a calendar rather than a stopwatch.

Don't take on an activity that is so time consuming it disrupts important schedules or obligations. An initial step to adding activity to your daily routine might be as simple as taking the stairs instead of the elevator or walking to the store instead of driving. When you make even modest changes, you create a starting point for your own motivation. In a few weeks or months, ask your spouse, other family member, or friend to join you in your routine. Having regular partners to train and talk with can make you healthier. Begin your new routine with fifteen or twenty minutes of moderate activity (or more, if you are in better shape).

My grandmother and I went for walks together while she lived with me. Although the pace was not quick enough for me to get an aerobic workout, it was effective enough for her to stay healthy well into her eighties. Our time together gave us many opportunities to share with each other. We would walk and talk while viewing a flower garden or stroking a neighbor's pet. At the age of eighty-two, she told me she wanted to start running! We began very slowly, with run segments of no more than twenty seconds each, mixed with three to four minutes of walking. Eventually she completed a five-kilometer (3.1 miles) race in just under forty-five minutes! She had a sense of pride in her accomplishment as she received a standing ovation for her athletic accomplishment. This is not to suggest that all octogenarians should enter a road race. Nor is it necessary to take up running as the only means to stay healthy. But if you are the kind of person who needs goals large or small to keep you going, don't hesitate to set some soon after you get started.

PRACTICAL IDEAS FOR GETTING STARTED

Perhaps you wonder how in the world you can fit another thing into your daily schedule. Instead of taking more of your time, good wellness habits actually extend the time you have. Here are some tips to help get you moving:

1. *Make a plan.* Keep an appointment with yourself to be active every day. This works well if you have a schedule that remains the same from week to week. If your schedule changes, sit down one evening and write your workout appointment into your schedule for the week. My brother Chris has made a lifetime commitment to fitness. He runs three times a week on his lunch break. He doesn't change this unless it is absolutely necessary. If he misses his midday workout, he knows he will have less time to spend with his daughters after work.

2. *Look for blank spots in your calendar.* Almost everyone can find fifteen to thirty minutes for exercise. For instance, I include exercise anytime I have my car worked on; I simply run or cycle home. Or I intentionally go out of my way to take an overnight package to a drop-off box fifteen minutes from my office. By fitting exercise into your daily schedule (like after taking children to school or seeing your spouse off to work), it becomes easier to stay consistent and build healthy patterns.

3. *Make an appointment to exercise with a friend.* Plan your week to include a friend or family member in an activity that you both enjoy. Many people are motivated by hav-

ing someone to work out with. Since most of us don't want to let an exercise partner down, we end up working out when we might otherwise stay in bed.

4. *Develop a time-line strategy.* World-class athletes develop a strategy that will carry them through three months, six months, or a year. Choose one or two goals that are realistic. The goal might be as simple as completing two laps on your favorite course or hiking a trail. Personal goals motivate you during moments when other priorities demand your attention. Once you reach a goal, reward yourself by backing off slightly—then set your sights on something new.

5. *Use a hard/easy system.* If you work out hard one day, take it easy the next. Give your body a chance to heal or repair itself after vigorous activity. Our bodies need more recovery time as we age. If you work toward a thirty-minute run/walk on Monday, Wednesday, and Friday, back off to fifteen or twenty minutes on Tuesday and Thursday. Or try a different activity, such as strength training, on the days between your aerobic efforts.

6. *Use variety to maintain your enthusiasm.* Do different activities and try new routes. Exercise with different people. Use exercise to go places you might not otherwise go. I use my daily walking, running, and cycling routes to take me to new neighborhoods, discover new trails, and explore the cities I visit.

7. *Make it fun for the entire family.* As your children get older (if they are still in the house), introduce them to a variety of activities. Experience new sports, activities, trails, or routes together.

8. *Hire a certified personal trainer.* A personal trainer will help
   you build a regular exercise pattern. Find a person with a
   degree in exercise physiology, exercise science, or a related
   field. A good trainer will instruct you how to exercise
   properly—pushing you without breaking you. Just as a
   tennis instructor can help you to learn the technique and
   rules of the game, a good personal trainer can teach you
   techniques and effective methods for maximizing your
   time and reaching your personal goals.

Choosing the Right Activities

Aerobic exercise should always be the cornerstone to your exercise
pattern. Aerobic means *in the presence of air.* In simple terms, the
level of oxygen available to you will meet the demands of your level
of activity. Aerobic exercise is any activity that uses your large
muscle groups for an extended period of time (twelve to twenty
minutes minimum). The following elements must be present to
produce a training effect:

- It must be continuous.
- It must use major muscle groups.
- It must be moderate enough so you are not gasping for
  breath or anaerobic (without oxygen).
- It should last between twelve and sixty minutes.

Activities such as walking, cycling, cross-country skiing, rowing, and swimming are examples of aerobic exercise. It is important, especially as we age, to warm up adequately before and to cool
down after any strenuous exercise. Start with three to ten minutes
of warmup to prepare your body to process the increasing levels of
oxygen—and to prepare for the increased workload. Once you

finish, allow time for a brief cool-down and for stretching. The cool-down gives your heart a chance to slow as your body temperature returns to normal.

Following are ten exercises and the calories each burns. The numbers are based on a 150-pound person exercising continuously for thirty minutes.

1. bicycling, vigorous (15 mph)   340 calories
2. jogging (10-12 minutes per mile) 340
3. swimming, vigorous   340
4. cross-country ski machine   323
5. spinning (indoor cycle)   312
6. jumping rope, slowly   272
7. tennis, singles   272
8. hiking, uphill   238
9. inline skating   238
10. walking, uphill (3.4 mph)   204[2]

Your First Three Months

As we get older, intensity should be replaced by consistency. This is one of the reasons I suggested earlier that you measure your progress with a calendar instead of a stopwatch. It is important, especially in the beginning, to enjoy what you do rather than dread it. This isn't to say intensity is always bad. But as we get older, our activity choices should reflect an improved health status instead of lowering our personal best in the marathon! To keep activity fun, don't overdo it. Take it slowly. If you increase intensity or length, do it in small stages.

There are several rules to keep in mind during the first three months of any new exercise program.

- As you complete an activity, you should always feel as if you could do more.
- Select an activity or sport that you are capable of doing over the long haul.
- Remember that seasonal sports are just that—seasonal. Choose an activity you can do all year long.

How can you know if you are exercising too hard? One way is to use the "talk test." That is, you should be able to engage in simple conversation during exercise. When the oxygen supply meets demand, you should be able to breathe comfortably. The harder you exert yourself, the more difficult it is to converse. The talk test is a simple, conservative way to monitor whether your workout is fun and whether your body is working efficiently to burn calories.

I recently took a day off while working in northern California to visit my sixty-one-year-old aunt. I don't remember her doing any physical exercise when I was younger. So I was pleasantly surprised when she suggested we go for a half-day ride on our mountain bikes. As we strapped on our helmets and positioned our bikes, I asked how long she had been riding. She explained she had done nothing to stay in shape until she began riding seven years ago. Now she was doing sixty-mile rides on the weekends! This stereotypically nonactive and out-of-shape woman descended the first hill with the grace, skill, and speed of someone far younger. When I asked her why she kept at the riding, she said, "I figured I better do something good for myself. Besides, I really enjoy it."

Enjoyment is key to exercising as we get older. For me, much of my enjoyment comes from the time I spend exercising with family and friends as I crisscross the country in my work in sports management. I have the closest relationships with people I have enjoyed running or cycling with in the past. Although the years have taken us to different cities or jobs, the common bond of mutual activity still unites us. When I am on the road, I try to schedule an overnight stop in those cities where I can see one of these friends. We run a local road race, hike a favorite trail, or bike together. This gives us the opportunity to get caught up on family life, kids, professional pursuits, or progress in our spiritual lives. It also provides an unspoken long-term accountability for continuing lifelong fitness patterns. Some of my most memorable moments are those spent with friends while enjoying an activity or hearty workout. The variety of activities and locations, as well as the relational aspects, make exercise more enjoyable.

THE STRUGGLE FOR CONSISTENCY

As a wellness coach, I work with fifty-six-year-old Mary Lou, a first-grade teacher I have trained for five years. I now meet with her once a week for a workout and instruction. During the walking phase of our workout, we talk about current goals, her health status, and what is happening in our lives. "I only walked once since I last saw you," she announced to me recently. I reminded her that the greatest weakness in any exercise plan is to be inconsistent. After watching hundreds of people succeed and fail with their exercise routines, I am now convinced that those who fail do so because they put too much pressure on themselves. They forget their personal purpose and forget that fitness must be a long-term commitment.

Always remain focused on *making exercise part of your lifestyle.* It is far more important to stay consistent than to work hard for several weeks or months and then quit. *Consistency is the most important and most neglected part of fitness for people of any age.* One reason people quit is because they get out of a healthy pattern. And any changes to the daily routine can distract you from a good habit. Travel, school holidays, vacation, and other changes in our routine can have an adverse effect on our physical well-being.

If you have ever struggled to stay consistent, here is a simple rule: Don't be afraid to allow yourself to miss two days of exercise, but never take off more than three or four days (unless you are injured). Think of your exercise routine as something you measure over the course of a month or year; from that perspective, a day or two off won't hurt. If you are faithful, you still will see and feel results.

Breaking Old Patterns and Overcoming Fears

For anyone who has ever started and stopped an exercise program, you understand how clever the excuses can be. Let's take a moment before we conclude this chapter to examine a few of these age-old excuses.

"It's too late to start." Just the opposite is true. It is never too late. The day you start is the day your body will begin to experience the benefits. No matter how old you are, what your ability or gender, or how fit (or out of shape) you are, your body needs activity. We each need a certain level of physical fitness to carry out everyday tasks.

"I have tried exercise, and I never seem to lose weight. Why should I waste my time?" You may not lose weight immediately. However, with consistent aerobic activity you *will* lose fat and increase your lean body mass. At approximately twenty minutes into an aerobic exercise session, your body shifts into what is called the "fat-burning phase," during which your body begins to burn fat as the primary source of energy. Once you have exercised beyond twenty

minutes, you burn more stored fat. An ideal program for weight loss is to exercise at a low or moderate intensity for thirty to sixty minutes, four to six times per week. You can participate in a strength-training program on alternating days that will help to increase muscle mass (which better equips us to burn fat).

"I need the right equipment to exercise." All you really need is a good pair of running or walking shoes; most people spend far more money on a suit or dress that hangs in the closet most of the year. As your level of fitness grows, reward yourself with a new piece of equipment, such as a dumbbell or running watch. Don't fall into the trap of believing you would exercise more if you only had a certain piece of equipment. While many people do use home exercise equipment, many let their expensive equipment serve as clothes hangers!

It comes as no surprise that getting started with an exercise program or routine after forty is more of a challenge than if we had established healthy patterns earlier in our lives. Still, whether we are in our forties or eighties, any increase in our activities (if it doesn't lead to injury) is bound to be beneficial to us. As Baby Boomers look to retirement and those over sixty start to retire, it becomes increasingly important to make physical activities part of our later years. The following chapter is designed to address ways to remain busy and active as we reach retirement age.

FOUR

Staying Busy After Retirement

DON OTIS AND LAURIE ELLSWORTH

There are very few things you can do to defy the aging process.
Keeping your hopes alive is definitely one of them.

—Dr. Stanley H. Cath

Tom Mason is fifty-seven years old and not entirely ready for retirement. Although he took early retirement, he immediately went on to become executive vice president of Focus on the Family. Tom likes to run and has done so since his midthirties. He runs three to five miles, four or five days a week. In the winter, he uses a treadmill; during the summer, he enjoys running outdoors. He says, "I am a believer that a healthful lifestyle can maximize the joy, quality, and productivity of whatever life span the Lord grants."

Planning and goal setting play an important role in what we decide to do after we retire. For Tom, one of his long-term goals has been to run in the Peachtree Road Race, one of the most prestigious road races in the country. He has successfully run in eighteen of the last nineteen races.

Developing both short- and long-term goals can keep you amply motivated well into retirement. No matter how old you are, you can set achievable goals. The Lilac Bloomsday Road Race held in Spokane, Washington, each year is the largest timed road race in the world. The twelve-kilometer race (7.4 miles) includes dozens of competitors who are over eighty years old! As Marvin Lloyd, an eighty-two-year-old competitor at the Georgia Golden Olympics, recently declared, "I'm not shooting to be running when I'm ninety. I'm shooting for one hundred!"

The number of people fifty-five and older who exercise regularly has grown 75 percent since 1987.[1] While remaining active plays a vital role in our health, healthy eating is also important as we get older. Tom visited the Cooper Clinic on two occasions for a full physical diagnostic checkup. One scan detected a high amount of calcification in his coronary artery. As a result, Tom made some adjustments in his diet. He now eats a diet high in vegetables, fruits, and carbohydrates and low in fat.

For this chapter I have enlisted the help of Laurie Ellsworth, a fitness educator, personal trainer, and college instructor. Her education in kinesiology and her expertise in working with senior adults is an invaluable contribution to understanding how we can remain active during retirement. Most important, she is a Christian who puts into practice the principles she discusses.

Reinventing Yourself

Peter Butler is sixty-eight years old. He didn't start running until he turned forty. Today Butler estimates that he has run four hundred marathons. "I have no thoughts of cutting back my running anytime soon," he says. "I hope to pursue my favorite hobby until I'm at least eighty."[2]

John Cahill is a seventy-five-year-old who didn't start to exercise until after his sixty-second birthday. He looked in the mirror and didn't like what he saw—an overweight, bored tax attorney. So he started running during a vacation and hasn't stopped. At first he couldn't finish a half-mile. Now he has run marathons, lost thirty pounds, and feels better. "The real benefit for me has been my health. I began to eat better and become tuned in to what my body wants and needs. My new lifestyle has also provided me with an activity to feel excited about in my advancing years."[3]

It is no secret that some men go downhill physically and emotionally shortly after retirement. Many find it difficult to adjust to a lifestyle in which they no longer feel productive. This is a tragedy that can be prevented. Retirement is not about doing nothing. It is about change. It is about doing something new. We can only imagine what the aging Moses must have felt when God called him to lead the Israelites out of Egypt at the ripe age of eighty! It wasn't until his "retirement years" that the work God had specifically called him to do was just getting started.

As Christians, retirement is a time to refocus or redirect our efforts. The new activities we participate in may be different from what we have been accustomed to doing. For many of us, like Moses, we may not know exactly what it involves.

The people who effectively navigate retirement are those who reach out to others. This means they get involved in social activities at church or in the community. Like eighty-three-year-old Evalyn, they volunteer to help others. She heads up the Alzheimer's support group in her community, mentors young people once or twice a year at Youth with a Mission bases, is active in visiting those who are sick, and does water aerobics. In addition, she works in a restaurant several days a week. In other words, she stays busy! This is the definition of a healthy retirement.

I struck up a conversation with seventy-five-year-old Ed in the gym one day. His leg was pockmarked with shrapnel wounds from a German mortar shell that landed next to him during World War II. The shell claimed one leg and left his remaining leg mangled. Still, during more than forty years of disability, Ed has always kept moving, riding a stationary bike and lifting weights to stay healthy. While retiring from a job requires making adjustments in one's daily routine, it should not be synonymous with inactivity. To the contrary, many active seniors actually become more physically active than they were during their working years.

A CHANGING LANDSCAPE

By the year 2010, the number of fifty-five- to seventy-four-year-olds will outnumber twenty-five- to thirty-four-year-olds by 18 million. The health industry—clubs, nutritional supplement manufacturers, and equipment suppliers—is gradually recognizing the changing marketplace. The $10-billion-a-year fitness industry is preparing for the senior fitness boom.

Tom Mason on the Retirement Myth

Retirement is one of the most misunderstood words in the language today. It is a relatively recent phenomenon and generally conjures up visions of golf fairways and sandy shores. There is an implication that we should back away from all real activity when we retire. Yet evidence shows that people who remain active and mentally engaged for a lifetime will live longer, healthier, and more productive lives. Physical activity is a part of this, but mental activity is equally important.

Someone has rightly said, "You should not retire *from* something, you should retire *to* something." There should be as much planning for the phase of life following a primary career as there was for the primary career itself. During an interview, newscaster Tom Brokaw once said that he planned to do network news for a few more years, and then it would be time for him to be "repotted." This is a great vision for the next stage of life—a time to be transferred to new soil, new activities, new challenges.

Most Americans no longer view life as linear. In times past, we went to school and then we worked. After that, we retired and did nothing. Today we go to school, work, go back to school, work in another field, pursue special interests, continue in school (or short-term equivalents), work in yet another field, and so on. Our path today is full of interesting diversions and direction changes.

Several years ago, at the age of fifty-two, I began attending weekend extension courses taught by Dallas Theological Seminary. I am now close to a master of biblical studies degree. It is not an education that I am pursuing for some career aim. Instead I simply desire to spend time studying subjects that interest me. One of the joys of approaching the end of a primary career is the opportunity to devote time and effort to the study of areas outside of a career field, subjects that simply interest us.

Likewise, the opportunity to contribute time and talent to pursuits and organizations (such as ministries and community groups) that are in line with the passion of our hearts, rather than simply those that produce an income, can be one of life's greatest blessings. One of the most important reasons for planning financially for the time following our primary career is to allow us to give back in an area that we truly care about without having to consider the financial implications of doing so.

There is a great Nike magazine advertisement that portrays an exhausted runner standing under a hot shower, recovering from a run he has just finished. The caption under the picture simply states, "Runs end, running doesn't." The idea that physical conditioning is something that only the young should pursue is a mistaken idea. In fact, the young actually require focused conditioning less than the old. A youthful body can overcome neglect and abuse far better than a person in middle age and beyond. It is sad to see professional athletes who spend years working out in the pursuit of physical strength and stamina, only to stop when their playing days end.

The keys to good health and optimum physical condition at any age are painfully simple and have not changed since the dawn of man. They are diet, exercise, and rest. In other words, lifestyle. As for the exercisers, we may have a desire to walk more and run less as we get older, or to bike instead of downhill ski. The type of activity is not as important as the commitment to some kind of regular physical exertion.

This, you may have recognized, is a recurring theme in this book. Obviously the earlier we begin to make healthful changes, the more benefits we will reap. There are more and more examples of men and women in their seventies and eighties who continue to run and ski and even compete in marathons or triathlons. The human body is a marvelous machine that can continue performing for a lifetime if proper maintenance and moderation are the cornerstones of a person's lifestyle.

The traditional health club environment can be intimidating for seniors. The typical gym caters to eighteen- to thirty-five-year-olds whose goals are most often to keep their bodies looking beautiful. This is rarely the case with seniors. Instead, most are looking for the strength and energy to continue doing the things they have always done—yard work, walking, driving, or working. Today some health clubs have opened separate areas for fifty-and-overs. And some suppliers are marketing equipment specifically to seniors. This trend will continue to grow as Baby Boomers race toward retirement age.

Fitness After Sixty

Steve Colwell is a sixty-seven-year-old certified fitness trainer. He teaches fitness classes in health clubs and speaks in retirement communities about healthy living. He refers to retirement as a double-edged sword. "There's plenty of time to do the things you've always wanted to do, but some seniors choose to mentally and physically check out of life. Part of successful aging is continuing to be involved and active." When Colwell thinks about retirement, he looks at it as a time of change but not a time to retreat from living. "Retirement from a job, yes, but not retirement from life."[4]

The benefits of exercising as we age are proven. Studies indicate that women between the ages of forty and sixty-five who get thirty minutes of vigorous exercise every day, even just a brisk walk, reduce their chances of having a stroke by as much as 30 percent. "The major public health problem in this nation is sedentary lifestyle," says Dr. JoAnn Manson, chief of preventative medicine at Brigham and Women's Hospital. "The benefits from exercise are seen rather quickly, so a woman who doesn't start exercising until later in life still has a chance to cut her risk of stroke. The earlier you develop good habits, the better," says Manson.[5]

The advantages of exercise are not just physical:

- Physical activity benefits mental functioning. A recent string of experiments found that exercise helps improve recovery time from brain injuries and can hold off mental declines associated with dementia and Alzheimer's.[6]

- Regular weight-bearing exercise—jogging, jumping rope, walking briskly, or lifting weights—can boost bone density 3 to 5 percent a year. Women who exercise benefit from stronger bones, which means their likelihood of getting osteoporosis is significantly less.[7]

- A recent study by Johns Hopkins University followed a group of people sixty-one to ninety-one during a six-month regimen of regular exercise. All of the patients began the program with chronic congestive heart failure. After a half-year of walking on treadmills and riding stationary bikes, they increased muscle strength and doubled their aerobic capacity. Researchers say their findings dispute the idea that some people are too old or too frail to enjoy the fruits of regular exercise.[8]

- Exercise allows people even eighty or ninety years old and living in nursing homes to become stronger and more independent. Physical activity is good for the heart, mood, and confidence. Older people who become more active have increased energy.[9]

The sad truth is that 70 percent of older adults are inactive. This inactivity is the major source of physical and mental deterioration.

- Regular exercise raises your heart rate and greatly reduces stiffening of the arteries. (Picture a supple rubber hose instead of one that has become stiff and brittle.)
- Stiff arteries are a major cause of high blood pressure, which can lead to heart disease and stroke.
- People who are physically active are less likely to develop adult-onset diabetes.
- Regular activity may lower the risk of intestinal bleeding in later life by 50 percent.
- Strength training or resistance training can make the bones stronger, improve balance, and increase muscle strength and mass.
- Stronger muscles ease the strain of arthritis pain.[10]

In the remainder of this chapter, fitness instructor Laurie Ellsworth provides practical help for older adults who need guidance for remaining active and healthy.

Staying Active and Keeping Well

We've probably all heard the clichés about exercise: "We rest, we rust." "Use it or lose it." "No pain, no gain." Even the Greek physician Hippocrates, in the fifth century B.C., first stated this very principle when he said, "All parts of the body which have a function, if used in moderation and exercised in labors thereby become healthy, well-developed, and age more slowly. But if unused and left idle, they become liable to disease, defective in growth, and age quickly.[11]

Conversely, those who continue to move today—still doing their own housework, grocery shopping, or gardening—will be more likely to move tomorrow. I teach a seniors' exercise class where the average age is eighty, but you'd never guess their age by looking at them or listening to them. They are actively participating in the lives of their families and friends, with exuberance and enthusiasm. Sure, they have their share of aches and pains, and morning stiffness often requires an aspirin or two for pain relief, but they don't let it stop them. They have maintained their ability to get around, take care of themselves, and play with their grandchildren as a result of their daily choice.

Choice, Change, and Commitment

If we want to take pleasure in our golden years and live them to the fullest, we must embrace the three general rules of choice, change, and commitment.

CHOICE

All action begins with a choice. Whether that action helps us or harms us, it always begins in our minds—with a thought. People have three different thoughts regarding their health: They choose to care for themselves, to indulge themselves, or to maintain the status quo. My goal as I age is to be able to play with my grandchildren, devote time to my hobbies, stay out of a wheelchair, and to live independently. To accomplish these goals I must make a few sacrifices along the way, including regular exercise and healthy eating. I choose health.

Several years ago while vacationing at my grandmother's house in Sun City, Arizona (a planned community for those fifty-five and up), I visited a nearby health club. I assumed that the activities there would be less than challenging for me, since I was younger than their usual clientele. Instead, I found people who were serious about staying in shape. I enjoyed an intense workout with an exercise leader twice my age.

Some people choose indulgence. They are unwilling to give up their second portions, decadent desserts, and inactivity. As they age, they think, "I've worked hard my entire life, and now I'm going to enjoy it. I deserve to treat myself by eating as much as I want and doing as little as I want." This choice is an invitation for disease. These people may eventually lose their freedom to do even simple movements, such as carrying a bag of groceries or walking up a long flight of stairs, and may actually end up enjoying life much less.

The third choice is complacency. Herbert V. Prochnow said, "There is a time we must firmly choose the course we will follow, or the relentless drift of events will make the decision." This is exactly what happened to my father. He started smoking at the age of sixteen. After he survived his first heart attack at the young age of forty-seven, we begged him to quit, to eat better, and to start a walking program. He agreed that such changes were important, but he never did change. Dad was fifty-two when he died of his third heart attack. He never lived to see any of his grandchildren. Those who do not choose healthy living exist in a survival mode. They don't see the connection between today's actions and tomorrow's health and happiness.

So what will your choice be? Will you choose health, embracing moderate eating and daily exercise? Or will you choose to indulge yourself today and put off thoughts about what tomorrow may bring? Or will you choose the status quo—a choice that seems to imply your health will remain exactly the same, but which often leads to a downward spiral into disease?

CHANGE

If you have decided it's time to choose health, then your next step is change. We have all tried to change our lifestyle at one time or another—how we eat, how we spend our leisure, how much we exercise. Although difficult, change is possible. It's never too late. As a personal trainer, I've seen many people over sixty who have successfully started and stayed with regular programs of physical activity. (Of course, you should consult with your doctor before you begin any exercise program.)

Because each of us is different, what works for one person may not work for another. Identify what you have tried in the past that did *not* work. Then choose a new activity with these three things in mind:

- *Discomfort.* If you are not emotionally comfortable in a par-ticular setting, such as water aerobics, spinning classes, or mall walking, there is probably a better alternative. I would add, however, that if you are new to regular exercise, you should expect a certain amount of apprehension at first. Give yourself ample time (two to four weeks) before deter-mining that it is not for you.

- *Disability.* Take into consideration any physical limitations you have before you can begin. For example, a recent client I trained had polio, which caused severe weakness in her legs. Putting her on the treadmill or bike would have been inappropriate, so we used a machine called the Biodex, which allowed her to use her arms for aerobic conditioning in a seated position.

- *Dollars.* Your exercise program should be affordable. What-ever activity you participate in should fit within your budget.

PLANNING FOR SUCCESS: ARE YOU READY?
One of the best ways to improve your level of fitness and health is to have a plan. When a client comes to me for advice on starting an exercise program, I begin by determining his or her physical ability and mental readiness. You can use the same method to determine which activities you should participate in. Here are the four categories I use to determine the level at which a person should begin:

- Level 1: complete functional capacity with no limitations or injuries, excited about workout

---

Affordable Fitness

You don't have to spend a fortune—or even one cent—to make the most of your workout time. Whether you are looking for fitness opportunities in a certain price range or are simply looking for something different to do, consider the following suggestions:

- Free: Walk on trails or in the mall (the only expense is good walking shoes); play tennis at a park; bike ride; lift weights (soup cans, books) with exercise programs on television.
- Nominal fees: Join the YMCA; sign up for park district exercise classes; look for low-impact or chair aerobic classes at churches.
- Moderate fees: Join a health club that offers plenty of options; purchase high quality home-exercise equipment (treadmill, hand weights); take exercise classes at a community college.
- Premium fees: Hire a personal trainer to design a program; invest in state-of-the-art home-exercise equipment.

- Level 2: complete functional capacity with no limitations or injuries, hesitant to try new things
- Level 3: limited functioning and mobility due to disease or injury, anxious to start exercising
- Level 4: limited functioning and mobility due to disease or injury, hesitant to move

Before you can change (or begin) your exercise pattern, determine which of the four levels best describes you.

Level 1

Level 1 people may participate in sports activities, including individual sports (walking, running, cycling, swimming), one-on-one sports (tennis, racquetball, squash, badminton), and team sports (basketball, volleyball, softball). Participating in sports can combine exercise with fun, friendly competition, and socialization.

Training for marathons may be fine for some folks, but the majority of us prefer a gentler, kinder sport such as walking, cycling, and swimming. Even a person at Level 1, who is in great health and mentally ready for a vigorous workout, should start with a twelve-week walking program *before* running. The body adjusts more readily to exercise if we begin gradually and add intensity as our muscles allow. It is never prudent to push yourself to do an activity you are not physically ready for, no matter how inspired you might feel.

Walking is the most popular exercise, the simplest to do, and the least expensive. If you have not been active, walking is a good way to start your exercise program. A good speed for someone at Level 1 is a seventeen-minute mile for two to three miles. Tip: Invest in good shoes and use walking trails through parks to enjoy nature.

Weight training is important for all fitness levels. You can start by purchasing one-, three-, five-, and eight-pound hand weights (or using soup cans of differing weights). You can also rent or purchase quality exercise videos such as The Firm Series or anything by Kathy Smith. Weight training should be done two to three times a week to maintain muscle mass, joint integrity, and a high metabolism. Tip: Work weaker muscles harder, such as the triceps (back of the arm), hamstrings (back of the upper leg), and upper back. By creating balance between opposing muscles, you'll help prevent injury and strengthen your joints.

Swimming is an excellent activity for complete conditioning, keeping your muscles strong and providing an aerobic workout. As a survival skill, swimming also allows you to participate with confidence in other recreational activities such as sailing, water skiing, canoeing, and scuba diving. If you didn't learn to swim as a child, it's not too late. Many people in their fifties and sixties take swimming lessons for the first time. Try all the strokes and alternate them every few laps. Swim for time rather than distance—shoot for twenty to thirty minutes. Tip: Learn to use a snorkel mask if you have trouble timing when to take a breath. Use goggles and a nose clip to protect your eyes and nose from the chlorine.

Running is one of the most challenging and efficient forms of aerobic exercise. It burns an extraordinary amount of calories per hour and raises your metabolism so you use more calories even in a state of rest. Running is safe when performed properly, starting slowly and working up to faster speeds and longer times. Begin your program with a goal of running fifteen minutes three times a week. Increase this time by five minutes per day every two weeks. Your final goal should be to run thirty minutes or more three times a week. Tip: Be sure to purchase a good pair of shoes and replace them before the cushioning wears out (about every five hundred miles) to avoid injury.

Flexibility is often the most neglected part of a fitness program, but it is even more important for seniors than for younger people. Over time, muscles shorten, particularly in the back, legs, and hips. This can cause injury during movement because the muscles are less pliable. Merv, a sixty-year-old client, shared this story with me: "I was helping my wife do some spring cleaning, and we were washing the windows. I leaned over a chair to open the window and felt a strange twinge across my back. I didn't think too much of it until the next morning. I could barely get out of bed. I've been in physical therapy for the last three weeks trying to get rid of the pain and loosen up my muscles." None of us wants to experience downtime—where we need rehabilitation to get better. That's why stretching before and after you exercise is so important, regardless what your level might be.

Level 2

People at Level 2 may be physically able to participate in all of the previously mentioned activities, but they are mentally unprepared (from fear of injury, pain, or not being able to finish) to work at the same intensity as Level 1. Level 2 people benefit most often from a walking program to build their confidence. As they experience success, they can advance to walking faster or increasing time—moving into Level 1.

Level 3

People at Level 3 may participate in all of the activities but at a low level of intensity and for a shorter time (based upon their physician's instructions). No one with limited mobility or the onset of disease should begin an exercise program without supervision. Once an exercise program is designed and completely understood, there is no reason a Level 3 person cannot continue exercise on her or his own.

Level 4
Level 4 is the category that most benefits from personal training or a physician-approved group exercise class. Once confidence is established and fears diminish (and this may take several months), a gentle walking program can be added as well, aiming at a thirty-minute mile.

Keeping the Commitment

Once we make the choice to begin an exercise program and change our activity level, we have to add one last ingredient for optimal health: commitment. Commitment is the willingness to stick with something even when we don't feel like it. Here are some ways to keep your interest long into your senior years:

- Use the buddy system. One of the greatest benefits of exercise is social. Working out with a friend is more fun, which means you will be more likely to repeat it.
- Vary your workout. Don't be afraid to try new activities. It will make exercising more interesting and challenging.
- Maintain an active lifestyle. Avoid too much television (more than an hour at a time), and participate in active hobbies such as dancing, gardening, golf, or woodworking.

Wherever you are in your quest, you can begin today with this commitment: *I will do what it takes to be healthy, and I will not give up!*

You will rarely find a chapter in any fitness book that deals with the mental aspects of eating right and exercise. As we have seen (and you undoubtedly know), healthy activities begin when our actions follow what our mind and will have determined is important. The reality is that many of us must deal with past failures or body-image issues before we can move forward into a healthy new lifestyle. In the next chapter Dr. Gregg Jantz helps us understand some of the issues that keep us from becoming healthier and offers solutions for what we can do about them.

FIVE

How the Mind Affects Fitness and Diet

GREGORY L. JANTZ, PH.D.

How you feel in your heart can show up in your body,
for your heart and body are more powerfully connected
than you have ever realized.

—DON COLBERT, M.D.

The human body spends a good deal of time on autopilot. Eyelids blink. Heart pumps. Glands secrete. Conscious thought just doesn't play a part. But there are aspects of our bodies in which conscious thought does play an enormous role.

Every bite we ingest, every liquid we swallow, every calorie we consume is deliberate. Every food choice is just that—a choice—and the choice is made in our minds. What is true for the food we eat is also true for the physical conditioning we establish. Physical conditioning and cardiovascular exercise are only accomplished under the control of the mind. If you decide to exercise, you will.

If you decide not to exercise, you won't. Of course, the mind is not entirely in the driver's seat, with the body merely going along for the ride; you may decide you are going to run a ten-kilometer (6.2 mile) race, only to have your body give out halfway.

Mind and body need to work in concert with each other in weight control and physical conditioning. Our thoughts, when birthed, produce feelings, and how we feel about something often dictates our actions. A sequence begins in the mind and results in actions by the body. If it is our goal to accomplish weight control and conditioning through proper food choices and exercise, it is important to understand the mind's role in helping or hindering our efforts.

All the Right Reasons

There are many reasons people decide to lose weight and exercise. Choosing the right reasons can help our efforts and contribute to our well-being. Right reasons are positive reasons. Positive reasons produce positive thoughts, which translate into positive feelings and positive actions. Let's turn our attention to some of these positive reasons for caring for the bodies God has given us.

BECAUSE GOD LOVES YOU

Nothing can be more positive than to know that God loves you. This is the core message of the gospel. God loves you and supports your decision to improve your health. He not only designed your body, He knows everything about it (see Psalm 139). God is and always has been solidly in your corner.

BECAUSE YOU LOVE GOD

As a Christian, you have committed your life to loving God through obedience to Him. As 1 John 5:3 says, "This is love for God: to obey his commands." Obedience to God is an appropriate and positive response to His love. It is wise to listen, therefore, when God speaks in His Word against misusing food through gluttony. And it is good to remember that "your body is a temple of the Holy Spirit, who is in you" (1 Corinthians 6:19). Physical fitness, then, can be viewed as a means of spiritual obedience. None of us would enter into a temple of God and trash His house. Living for God and dying to self is a wonderful motivation to treat His temple, your body, with respect and care through proper nutrition and exercise.

BECAUSE YOU LOVE YOURSELF

Jesus made an interesting statement. He said that we are to love our neighbors as ourselves (Matthew 22:39). Similarly, in the book of Ephesians, God says that husbands should love their wives as they love their own bodies (5:28). These commandments from God presuppose that we actually do love ourselves. Loving yourself and your body is a wonderful motivation and a positive reason for choosing a healthy lifestyle.

BECAUSE YOU LOVE OTHERS

Christians are called "the body of Christ." We become His outstretched hands and encircling arms. In order to join God in His work, we must be able—both spiritually and physically. Compassion and rendering aid require effort, often physical effort. The desire to be ready like Samuel and say, "Here am I" (1 Samuel 3,

KJV) is a powerful reason to keep yourself physically ready to respond to the needs of others, thus giving glory to God.

Positive reasons, stemming from God's love and radiating outward, provide the proper foundation for any decision to control weight and become more physically fit. These reasons strengthen our resolve to begin, cushion us when we become discouraged, and encourage us when we need to commit anew. But as we know, this world is made up of both the positive and the negative. Our resolve to maintain a healthy lifestyle is affected by both kinds of influence. While striving to operate from a positive mental position, we should be aware of the adverse effects of negative thinking.

Wrong Voices, Wrong Reasons

Love is a powerful and positive motivator to action and changed behavior. Not every powerful motivator is positive, however. Since we are people surrounded by sin and the consequences of sin, negative reasons and the thoughts, feelings, and actions they produce can also be powerful. For many, these negative factors rise more quickly to the surface than their positive counterparts. Satan is also a deceiver. He will attempt to make negative reasons appear to be good reasons. Only through keeping our eyes on Christ can we understand the truth behind our desires and motivation to lose weight and keep fit.

Love for the World

While love for God should be a positive motivation in lifestyle changes, too often love for the world is a negative one. Our culture credits outward appearance over inner beauty. Our culture values instant results, not patient persistence. Many of us listen too much to the world and not enough to God when we are making decisions regarding a change in our lifestyle. We look in the mirror and see only the negative subtraction of youth and not the positive addition of age. We want to look as good as, or better than, we did "back then." We look at worldly views of beauty and strength and decide we're running out of time to achieve them. We become angry and frustrated when each passing year makes us "older and wider."

Such anger can energize us in our initial resolve to begin a nutrition or exercise program. But this hot flash of anger can, over time, debilitate instead of empower. Anger can lead to pessimism, and pessimism can lead to fatalism. Fatalism smothers the positive motivation of hope and dooms many lifestyle changes to failure. Disgusted with ourselves, we give up and return to our previous food behaviors to give us comfort. Not only do we return to our unhealthy choices, we further degrade ourselves physically through additional weight gain.

Even when this anger is viewed as a positive motivator in eating patterns and exercise, it can have unexpected negative repercussions. It can fuel a view of the body as an enemy to be punished and controlled. It can contribute to the idea that food is an adversary to be controlled and conquered. This path of anger can appear to have a successful beginning because of actual weight loss, but too often it ends in disaster.

HATRED OF SELF

God has always intended for us to love ourselves and to live a positive life in Him. Unfortunately, some people hate who they are and how they look. They look in the mirror and see ugliness staring back at them. Self-hatred can fuel a desire to punish the body for its perceived betrayal of being overweight and growing older.

This negative reaction to our own bodies can be strengthened by patterns of thinking developed during childhood. Negative messages received as we were growing up have a way of adding to our own negative mental chorus whenever we attempt to make positive changes in our behavior as adults.

Over time these negative messages, both our own and those we have heard from others, produce a burden some find difficult to bear as they try to lose weight and eat right. Each sedentary day and every fast-food meal along the way produce a tremendous amount of guilt, which can provoke an inappropriate response. Either the guilt increases the self-loathing that leads to an eating disorder, or the guilt saps the resolve to continue and causes people to quit in frustration.

IMAGE IS EVERYTHING

We live in a world where youth and beauty are prized, where an overweight body is ugly and being slender is beautiful. We live in a society in which physical accomplishments define value. For women over forty, living with this image can be difficult when ideal women are usually younger and almost certainly thinner. Just look at the models who stare out at us from the glossy magazines in the checkout line at the grocery store. For men, in a world where most male heroes are athletes, the pressure is to maintain physical vigor and athletic prowess. These attributes translate into acceptance and approval from society at large. As we look at our bodies and compare them to the images emphasized in our culture, we invariably fall short.

The expectations of our culture, our peers, and ourselves can be at war with the reality of how we look and feel. Overwhelming feelings of guilt and inadequacy are often expressed by those unable to control their food choices or weight. It is unfortunate when a decision to improve your health mutates into a physically damaging compulsion. Guilt can also trigger or deepen depression. In the midst of depression, the strength and resolve to make healthy choices wither. In an effort to find comfort, we turn to food as a substitute, and the need to find inappropriate comfort through food increases the threat of compulsive eating behaviors. It is a tragedy when a decision to improve health degenerates into behaviors that actually endanger it!

Even as we review these negative voices in our lives, I cannot emphasize enough the need to embrace the positive when making a decision regarding lifestyle changes. Positive, godly reasons should be the platform upon which you build your commitment to a healthier lifestyle. Beginning with a positive attitude about nutrition and exercise is a hedge against the inevitable negative influences bound to crop up as you work toward integrating these healthy choices in your life.

Keeping Fit Wisely

Just as we need to decide to make healthier lifestyle choices for the right reasons, we also need to *maintain* those healthier lifestyle choices. The challenge is remaining positive when it seems that everything you do has a negative connotation in that you're having to "give up" something. Nutrition and exercise, in order to be properly maintained, must be viewed as a benefit to the quality of your life, not a detraction from it. They must be seen as positive, ongoing, and progressive steps toward health and wellness.

Down on Diets

The word *diet* has come to mean the food we don't eat rather than the food we choose to consume. That is why I tend to avoid the word. Diets are often short-lived and rarely successful. Often the most attractive aspect of the latest fad diet is how quickly it can be accomplished.

My experience has been that those who are successful losing weight on a diet end up gaining even more weight back once the diet is over. I have known many people whose weight has yo-yoed up and down the scale for years as a result of dieting, with weight gain winning out over the long haul.

Taking the Long View

It has been said that the longer it takes for you to lose weight, the longer you will successfully keep it off. *Quick diets produce quick results with quick relapses.* In order to maintain the positive outlook so vital to successfully integrating healthier lifestyle choices, it is important to view such choices as progressive and long-term. This isn't about dieting and sweating and denying your body for a week or a month. It's about eating and exercising and supporting your body for the rest of your life.

By the time you reach forty or older, you've spent a lot of time developing behavioral patterns that are now part of your life. This is especially true with eating habits and activity levels. It takes time and energy to correct these patterns. It takes prayer and perseverance. Only through remaining positive and upbeat about these changes can you find the motivation to continue with them. View the changes as if you were on a journey; they will take as long as necessary for you to reach your destination.

Facing the Fear

Many people find their motivation eroded by a trickle of fear that slowly eats away at their positive choices. They fear failure. This is especially true if the person has tried to eat right and exercise before—and failed. Failure the last time cries out against any hope of success the next time. If their past is littered with a string of failures, any momentary lapse in their current resolve is seen as proof they will fail again.

When fear of failure saps your strength to continue, face your fear head-on. Most of our fears and concerns are out of proportion to the actual events. Ask yourself, "What am I really afraid of?" Allow yourself to examine any deeper issues, or other voices, complicating your desire to live a healthier life. What are those other voices telling you? Where do they come from? What are they really saying to you about yourself? If they are negative, discard them! Drown them out with positive messages about yourself.

If you have trouble coming up with positive messages on your own, turn to Scripture. God's Word is full of encouraging messages about His love and forgiveness, about how He views you as His beloved child, about how His Spirit is within you to help and guide you.

The Power of Forgiveness

When did we forget the wisdom "If at first you don't succeed, try, try again"? A failure in the past does not doom our current efforts, unless we decide it will. Along the journey toward better nutrition and physical fitness, bumps in the road are bound to occur. Going over a bump while driving may jostle you and cause you to slow down, but it doesn't make you stop and turn around. There are stretches in the road of life where more bumps are bound to occur, usually during times of stress. There is nothing wrong, during these times, with slowing down as long as you continue to move forward.

Even if you have a backward lapse, this doesn't mean you must stop altogether. Instead, forgive yourself.

Forgive yourself, and resist the temptation to think fatalistically, to believe that a lapse means you should discard your whole regimen.

Forgive yourself, and resist the temptation to belittle yourself for your failure, replaying negative messages from your past.

Forgive yourself, and grab hold of God's grace. Don't dwell on the negative consequences of your lapse. Instead focus on the positive benefits you'll experience if you keep going.

FILLING THE RIGHT HUNGER

Scripture says that it is possible to eat and not be satisfied (Leviticus 26:26). But how can that be? If we fill up our stomachs with food, how can we not be satisfied? The answer to that question is one of the leading reasons people fail to maintain healthy food choices. We eat and are not satisfied because the hunger we are attempting to fill with food isn't physical. It isn't really about food at all. Food is being used to fill the void of loneliness, rejection, fatigue, stress, abuse, boredom. Food is being substituted for affection, affirmation, approval, comfort, even love.

The extremes of this behavior constitute what are known as eating disorders. I have found that a large number of people who would not be considered to have eating disorders, nevertheless use food for something other than physical nutrition. They may not binge and purge, but they do use food to reward, calm, or comfort themselves. For many, it is this stubborn mind-set that has sabotaged their best efforts to improve their eating habits.

It wouldn't be quite so hard to stick to healthy eating choices if most of us were likely to choose carrot sticks or apple slices as comfort food. Instead, it is usually something full of sugar, fat, or simple carbohydrates. And it wouldn't be so hard to stick to healthy eating choices if the comfort we sought was merely the comfort of relieving physical hunger. Instead, emotional hunger compels us to eat unwisely long after physical hunger has been satisfied. Negative thoughts arising from an emotional void propel our feelings of need. These feelings are then inappropriately translated into actions involving food. To maintain our healthy eating choices, we need to separate what we eat physically from how we feel emotionally.

This misdirection of food and comfort often occurs first during childhood, from patterns passed down to us from our parents. How many times did some of us hear, "Why don't you eat something? You'll feel better!" When we had a bad day or sustained a minor injury, how many times were we offered something sweet to take our mind off of it? How many times was good behavior rewarded by a treat? Is it any wonder, then, that as adults we turn to food for reasons other than physical hunger? Is it any wonder that we turn to less-than-healthy foods to fill us up?

In order to maintain healthy choices, food must be returned to the realm of nutrition instead of comfort. Ultimately we must look to God to fill the emotional voids in our lives. He gave us food to fill us physically. He gives us His Spirit to fill us emotionally and spiritually. It is His desire for us to look to Him—and not to food—for the inner comfort we so desperately seek. After all, He is called "the God of all comfort" (2 Corinthians 1:3). It is our relationship with Him that is to provide us with emotional comfort and fullness. When this happens, food can again take its proper place as the nutritional basis for our physical well-being. With this concept firmly planted, carrot sticks and apple slices can actually become comfort food, as we are comforted that God has supplied us with healthful food and the knowledge of healthy eating.

ALL PAIN, NO GAIN

A healthy lifestyle isn't restricted to what we put in our mouths. It includes physical activity as well. Negative influences don't just infiltrate our desire to eat healthfully; they also can complicate our resolve to exercise properly. Too often, physical activity is viewed negatively, as a punishment to be endured, as penance for the sins of a sedentary life. This negative approach will not provide the motivation we need to make exercise a regular part of our lives over the long haul.

When most of us think of exercise, we tend to think of the bulging muscles, dripping sweat, furrowed brows, and grunts of exertion found on a running track or in a gym. For some folks, that *is* fun. But for many people, it seems like an awful lot of dreary work. So they avoid it. But because they avoid it, they feel guilty. Because they feel guilty, they seek comfort. The comfort they go back to is often the comfort of food. It's an unproductive and unhealthy cycle.

Exercise must be viewed as a positive, enjoyable activity. Choose an activity you enjoy doing. As I wrote in *21 Days to Eating Better*, "Exercise must be something fully compatible with you and your personality."[1] The ways you can increase your physical activity level are myriad, from formal sports activities to working around your house or taking your dog for a walk.

The first thing you try might not work as well as you'd like. Don't be discouraged! Try something else, or add to what you're already doing. Look at your day-to-day activities and find ways to build upon or enhance them. Be creative about finding ways to increase your physical activity level. Use some of the wisdom you've gained over the years to your advantage! It may not be just a matter of working harder but smarter as well.

THE POWER OF TWO

We have talked about the negative implications of coupling comfort with food. There are some positive implications, however, of coupling two other things: fitness and camaraderie.

In Christian circles many people have found value in an "accountability" group. This is a group of individuals who come together to encourage one another in a common goal, usually striving toward greater spiritual maturity. This is a concept that can also assist people in their journey toward a healthier life. Ecclesiastes 4:12 states the concept this way: "Though one may be overpowered, two can defend themselves. A cord of three strands is not quickly broken." An Indiana University study reinforces this timeless biblical truth. The study found that couples who exercise together were seven times as likely to stick with their fitness programs as subjects who were partnerless.[2]

When a group or partnership is formed, there is emotional bonding and accountability. For example, you might be tempted to forgo exercising on a given day. Maybe you're tired or it's raining or you just plain don't want to. If you are working with other people toward a joint goal of exercise and fitness, you may go ahead and exercise even when you don't want to, rather than have a negative effect on them. And even though you are initially participating for others' sake, many people find that they end up benefiting themselves. In other words, they think they are too tired, but after walking around the park with a friend or group, they feel energized and happier.

There is another positive benefit of people's exercising together. They realize they are not alone. Isolation can produce negative thoughts and depression. By working with a group of people who are in a similar situation and united in goals, isolation is turned into commonality and shared strength. When one falters, another can provide relief. When one excels, another can take courage. Just as God formed us together as a church to support each other spiritually, a group can provide the support we need to begin and maintain our healthy choices.

How the Body Gives Back to the Mind

Thoughts, feelings, and actions work from the mind to the body, but the connection doesn't end there. While positive thoughts can translate into physical benefits, physical activity can return the favor: Exercise can reduce the negative effects of stress. Personally, I can attest to the value that exercise plays in my own life, especially in preparing me to handle the stress of living my life and running my business.

According to Dr. Michael Steelman, past president of the American Society of Bariatric Physicians, who specialize in weight-related issues, even modest weight loss can give people an emotional boost. "It gives them the kind of self-confidence they need to move ahead with their life, perhaps to earn promotions, to change jobs, to improve relationships," he says. The energizing feeling of success in a healthy lifestyle can open up the possibility of success in other areas.

In our fast-paced, hectic society, stress not only degrades our health, it also batters our emotional stability. By lessening the negative effects of stress, exercise appears to bolster our ability to stay positive. A positive outlook in turn bolsters our resolve to exercise. This is the cyclical model of a successful, long-term pattern of a healthy lifestyle.

When More Is Needed

As a Christian counselor, I am aware that situations arise to complicate even the best efforts to maintain a healthy lifestyle. You may have chosen to read this book because you have an established pattern of trying and failing at different types of weight-loss plans over many years. You are aware of the passage of time and are afraid you will be doomed to live a life consumed by food and weight.

Your inability to eat and exercise healthfully may not be a question of having enough will power, enough faith, or enough friends to accomplish your goals. For you, it may be more than merely finding the right weight-loss or exercise plan. You may be suffering from an eating disorder or clinical depression. Both conditions will interfere with your ability to make responsible choices about the food you eat and your activity level. If you think you may have an eating disorder, seek out a caring Christian professional who can assist you in disconnecting food from inappropriate emotions and feelings. Learning the true reasons you turn to food can help you unlock unhealthy eating behaviors. A trained counselor can help you learn to love and respect your body, allowing you to view yourself positively and be motivated to treat yourself in an appropriate, godly way.

Clinical depression can also have a negative impact on eating patterns as well as activity levels. Depression robs you of the will to improve, to move, even the will to function at more than a basic level. Clinical depression is not just feeling down for a day or a week. And it is not something you can wish yourself out of. You will need to seek advice and receive support from a health professional on a method of treatment for this type of depression. If your ability to maintain a positive outlook on life has been seriously affected over an extended period of time, without relief, you may be suffering from severe depression. This will need to be addressed either prior to, or as part of, any decision to make healthy, positive lifestyle changes.

There is no shame in seeking out the help of others to assist you. Beware of the negative effects of shame and pride. Fight against the smothering effects of depression and lethargy. These lead to bondage to unhealthy choices and hidden hungers. Concentrate on the positive effects of confession and honesty. These lead to truth and freedom. They will enable you to make positive, life-affirming changes for your good. After all, our life, Jesus says, is more important than food (Matthew 6:25). Isn't it time we started living that way? The answer for me and for you can be a resounding "Yes!"

We have looked at motivation issues related to diet and exercise. We have also explained the many benefits of exercise and how to start making healthy lifestyle choices. Those of us who are over forty have already discovered that our bodies don't respond the way they did in earlier years. As we become more active, we also run the risk of injury. While injuries at any age can and do slow us down, some injuries can be avoided as we age. Others take special attention or treatment. In the next chapter, Dr. Andrew Seddon describes some of the most common injuries and how to avoid them.

SIX

Aging, Exercise, and Injuries

ANDREW M. SEDDON, M.D.

Exercise improves posture, reduces dysfunction of the joints and strengthens the bones.

—FRANCISCO CONTRERAS, M.D.

"Bodily exercise profiteth little," according to the *King James Version's* translation of the apostle Paul's word in 1 Timothy 4:8, apparently dismissing physical fitness at a stroke. Modern translations soften his words ("bodily training is of some value," RSV), but the impression remains that he was unconcerned with toning mere flesh. He was comparing the body and the spirit ("spiritual fitness is of unlimited value," Phillips), a limited physical life versus an eternal spiritual existence.

In Paul's time the contrast seemed even greater than in our own day. The average first-century citizen could expect to live some thirty or forty years, at the mercy of Roman military action (if Jewish or barbarian), barbarian military action (if Roman), plagues, malnutrition, and natural disasters—many of the same factors that still limit life expectancy in large areas of the world. But in our ever-more-affluent early-twenty-first-century Western society, life expectancy for both men and women has reached the upper seventies.

With our longer life expectancy comes maladies unknown to or rare in the ancient world. We are plagued by diseases of aging—cancers, coronary artery disease, cerebrovascular disease, Alzheimer's disease, the complications of diabetes, and many others. Because of this, physical fitness assumes a greater importance for us than for first-century humans. Fitness helps maintain health and prevent or ameliorate the effects of age-associated disease. It's actually riskier *not* to exercise.

Maybe if Paul had been given that choice, he'd have been more encouraging about the state of our bodies.

Know What You're Up Against

While it's undoubtedly an exaggeration to claim that "life begins at forty," we can safely conclude that it doesn't *end* then. Consider Gordie Howe suiting up for the National Hockey League at age fifty-two; Ashley Harper swimming the English Channel at sixty-five; Richard Bass reaching the summit of Mount Everest at fifty-five; Nolan Ryan pitching no-hitters in his forties. While most of us over-forties aspire to more modest goals than Wimbledon or Masters' titles, we *can* stay active. But we have to realize that our bodies do change, aging in ways that are largely related to our genetic design. Like it or not, we're not twenty-year-olds any longer.

Maximal heart rate (220 minus age) declines and limits cardiac output and maximal aerobic capacity. Reduced kidney function leads to difficulty in controlling fluid volumes and electrolytes. The lungs (and associated muscles and chest wall structures) lose effectiveness, particularly if they've been damaged by smoking, pollutants, or infections. Blood vessels harden and narrow. Nerve conduction velocities slow, coordination diminishes, and reflex times increase. Bones thin, connective tissue wastes and loses tensile strength, cartilage degenerates, and muscles stiffen and weaken.

In short, our hearts can't pump like they used to through blood vessels that increasingly resemble copper pipes; our kidneys need tender loving care to keep us from bloating into watermelons or withering into prunes; our lungs can't deliver as much oxygen as they should to muscles that resemble old rubber bands; our brains can't get us to move like we used to; and if by some miracle we get it all together, we still have creaky bones and rusty joints to contend with.

Not a pretty picture. It's almost enough to make us abandon exercise all together and join our lazy techno-society in reaching for the video remote. Right?

Wrong! Exercise can improve the functional capacity of all body systems. In fact, regular exercise may retard the physiologic decline associated with old age by as much as 50 percent.[1] Our bodies are designed to function better with exercise. We can't join the 15 to 50 percent of people who are sedentary, the one-third of men and two-thirds of women who would find it hard to sustain a moderate walk,[2] or contribute to the depressing statistic that the average American is heavier now than in 1980.[3]

The benefits of exercise are worth the risks. But how do we go about exercising safely? By using our brains. We must tailor our exercise program to our individual needs, goals, and physical state.

What do you want to accomplish? Do you want to exercise for fun? To lose fifty pounds? To lower your cholesterol? To win the state tennis championship for your age bracket? To climb

Mount Kilimanjaro? Be sensible and realistic. Your goals will largely determine the specific activities you choose, which will, in turn, determine the potential for injury. Current recommendations are for thirty minutes of moderate exercise most days of the week. Briskly walking as little as one and a half to two miles three times a week will have beneficial effects.

Know Your Body

Age-related changes in body systems occur in everyone, but not at the same rate. One person might have strong bones, but a bad heart. Another might have good lungs, but poor kidneys. It is crucial to know your own body—its strengths and weaknesses, its capacity, its potential for improvement, and its vulnerabilities. There's no escaping the consequences of the accidents and mishaps that attended our growing years; they've contributed to the current state of our bodies. Knowing how we are *now*—not how we used to be—puts us on the road to safe exercise.

Talk with your personal physician. A physical examination can't guarantee that you won't get hurt, of course, but in many cases it can show your specific physical risks. The American Academy of Family Physicians (AAFP) suggests, "Because the risks of activity are very low compared with the health benefits, most adults do not need medical consultation or pretesting before starting a moderate-intensity physical activity program. However, a medical evaluation should be performed in people with cardiovascular disease and in men over forty and women over fifty years of age with multiple cardiovascular risk factors who contemplate beginning a program of vigorous activity."[4] (Cardiovascular risk factors include smoking, obesity, hyperlipemia, family history of heart disease, high blood pressure, and diabetes.) As we'll see, though, paying attention to physical condition may be more important than the AAFP indicates.

Specific areas that may be targeted in an examination include:

- *The cardiovascular system.* Evidence of coronary artery disease (which becomes more common over forty, particularly in men), heart rhythm abnormalities, heart enlargement, high blood pressure, or poor circulation in peripheral arteries and veins may be detected. Cardiovascular problems don't preclude exercise, but they may require alterations in the level or type of activity or require preactivity treatment. Specific testing (such as an exercise stress test) may be suggested in specific instances.

- *The metabolic system.* Diseases such as diabetes, thyroid disorders, and electrolyte imbalances may not have obvious symptoms but can have severe effects. Metabolic disorders are detected in blood screening tests.

- *The nervous system.* Changes in coordination and balance may influence the safety of various activities.

- *The respiratory system.* Adequate oxygen exchange is crucial to exercise. Many conditions affect lung functioning. Exercise-induced asthma is a common cause of sports-related respiratory difficulty.

- *The musculoskeletal system.* The bones, muscles, and joints take the brunt of exercise and injury. Despite a common misconception, there is no data to support the belief that exercise contributes to the development of arthritis.

One easily overlooked potential source of complications lies in medications, both prescribed and over-the-counter. It's easy to forget that certain high blood pressure medicines (beta blockers) can slow the heart rate and diminish exercise capacity; antidepressants can cause dizziness, impair sweating and the body's heat-control mechanisms that lead to heat-related injury (heat exhaustion and sunstroke); antihistamines and antianxiety medications can cause drowsiness and slow coordination; medications for diabetes can lead to hypoglycemia; diuretics can affect kidney function and lead to dehydration and electrolyte abnormalities.

Does that mean we should abandon all medications before exercising? Absolutely not! Common sense says we shouldn't stop taking any medication prescribed for a chronic condition without our doctor's approval. (Stopping some medicines abruptly can have serious consequences.) But the effects of medications need to be considered when planning exercise regimens. Medications don't have to pose barriers to exercise, but they must be factored into the equation.

In summary, know as much as you can about your body. Listen to what it is telling you. Tailor your activity to your physical condition, and choose the most appropriate exercise. Never exercise before any unusual or worrisome symptoms have been explained (or determined to be harmless) to the best of your physician's ability.

Know Your Sport

Once you've been cleared for exercise and you've decided on an activity, the next step is to know your sport. Once again, there's no substitute for thoughtful preparation. Medical offices treat legions of injured "weekend warriors" who have launched into aggressive exercise without proper preparation and knowledge of their sports.

Know the risks of your particular sport. Know what training is required. Know the preparation needed, whether it's nutrition, hydration, stretching, or strengthening. Acquire any recommended protective equipment—there's a reason for it—and obtain the right equipment for the sport. Both technique and equipment can make a great difference; cutting corners can hurt. Local athletic clubs, fellow enthusiasts, and professional sports trainers can provide information.

Any activity should be preceded by preparation. Don't play cold. An appropriate warmup might consist of ten to fifteen minutes of static and slow stretching of major muscle groups, then five minutes of low-level calisthenics, then a few minutes of sports-specific activity at a low level. Be certain you're hydrated, that your nutrition is adequate, and that you're dressed appropriately for the environmental conditions.

Popular Sports and Their Most Common Injuries

Basketball
Ankle sprain, Achilles tendon rupture, shin splints, knee injuries, head trauma, calf muscle strain and tear, patellar tendinitis (jumper's knee), finger injuries, eye injuries

Cycling
Back and neck pain, head injury, abrasions (road rash), contusions, lacerations, upper and lower extremity fractures, patellar tendinitis, iliotibial band friction syndrome, ulnar nerve compression, pudendal neuropathy in male cyclists

Golf
Lateral epicondylitis (golfer's elbow), back sprain

Racquetball
Eye injuries, facial and nasal injuries, also see Tennis

Running
Shin splints, stress fractures, sprains, tendinitis, patellar problems, plantar fasciitis

Skiing
Knee injuries, frostbite, altitude sickness, hypothermia, sun exposure (skin and eyes), skier's thumb

Soccer
Head injury, concussion, exertional headache, neck strain, groin strain

Swimming
Shoulder tendinitis and bursitis (swimmer's shoulder), breast-stroker's knee, back and neck pain, dermatological conditions, ear infections, conjunctivitis, drowning

Tennis
Lateral epicondylitis (tennis elbow), shin splints, back sprain, Achilles tendon rupture, shoulder tendinitis and bursitis, anterior cruciate ligament tear

Weightlifting
Muscle strains, thoracic outlet syndrome, shoulder impingement syndromes, acromioclavicular joint strain, disk herniations, weight-lifter's headache

Know the Injuries

Unfortunately injuries can occur to even the best-trained and prepared athlete. Most of these injuries are musculoskeletal.

Age makes a difference in the types of injuries that can be anticipated. Five components are needed for good physical performance: strength, endurance, speed, coordination, and flexibility.[5] All of these decline with age. While younger athletes experience higher rates of traumatic ligament and tendon injuries, due to their participation in more violent sport and the heightened intensity of their exercise, degenerative tissue problems are more common in older enthusiasts—the wear and tear resulting from chronic overuse or the accumulated trauma of years.

Not surprisingly, competitive sports pose higher risks than recreational activity, and contact sports are more hazardous than noncontact activities. Often it is not the level of activity that contributes to injury, but the repetition and frequency. Injuries can be precipitated by intrinsic factors (such as decreased flexibility) and extrinsic factors (training errors).

Injury results from a "simple mismatch between stress on a given tissue and the ability of that tissue to withstand the stress."[6] This can occur from macrotrauma—a single traumatic event that suddenly overwhelms a tissue and is usually noticed immediately by the athlete (like a sprained ankle), or it can result from microtrauma—a repetitive, overuse activity that gradually overcomes a tissue's healing ability (like tennis elbow or a stress fracture). Either can occur in any sport, but some sports are more likely to cause one or the other type.

The exact incidence of overuse injuries is not known, but it is estimated at 35 to 65 percent of all sports injuries.[7] The prevalence is certainly high enough that some authorities recommend an examination to identify weaknesses and flexibility defects to prevent overuse injuries.

Overtraining is a risk for the athlete determined on higher performance who wants results too quickly. It's simply not possible to go from a two-mile jog in the morning to trying to win the Boston Marathon a week later. Having an age- and condition-appropriate training regimen can be crucial to success. Keeping an exercise log may help motivation as well as reduce the risk of overtraining. Short-term symptoms of overtraining (such as fatigue, decreased competitive drive, and poor performance) may respond to a few days' rest, but longer-term complications require prolonged rest. Athletes who don't recognize the symptoms of overtraining risk chronic overuse injuries, failed performance, illness, and premature retirement from their sport.

PHYSICAL SIGNS OF OVERTRAINING

The following are signs that an athlete is overtraining and risking injury:

- increase in morning resting heart rate
- disturbed sleep patterns
- inadequate caloric intake with excessive weight loss
- increased thirst
- reduced performance capacity
- muscle soreness
- mood swings (decreased libido, decreased vigor, increased fatigue, depression, anger)
- "heavy," painful muscles
- depressed immune function

- loss of menstruation
- decreased competitive drive
- gastrointestinal disturbances (diarrhea)[8]

It's normal when beginning exercise to experience muscle soreness, tenderness, and stiffness. But how can this be distinguished from signs of overuse? There are three types of muscle soreness. Delayed soreness is the most common. It occurs twelve to forty-eight hours after exercise and it seems to be related to unbalanced muscle activity. Acute soreness occurs during activity, resolves with rest, and results from inadequate circulation to the affected muscles. Injury-related pain occurs during high-speed repetitive exercise and is similar to a pulled muscle.

COMMON INJURIES AND THEIR TREATMENTS
Let's look at some of the more common injuries resulting from macrotrauma and microtrauma.

The Foot
Our feet respond to trauma with bunion deformities, corns, and calluses. Metatarsalgia is pain and inflammation at the ends of the long bones in the foot; it responds to rest, anti-inflammatory medications, and improved footwear. Plantar fasciitis is inflammation of the connective tissues of the foot where they connect to the heel; treatment involves ice, stretches, anti-inflammatories, heel cups, and, possibly, corticosteroid injection.

Stress fractures are most commonly (but not exclusively) encountered by runners, particularly if they have increased the length and duration of running in preparation for a long race or marathon. Initial x-rays may show nothing out of the ordinary, and occasionally a bone scan or CT scan is needed to locate the fracture. A stress fracture is treated with rest and immobilization. The presence of either acute or chronic pain over the bones of the foot indicates the need for evaluation.

The Ankle

Strains and sprains typically occur over the lateral malleolus (the outside) and result from twisting the foot. Sprains and strains are graded as:

Grade I: mild, microscopic tears in tissue fibers
Grade II: moderate, partial disruption of tissue structure
Grade III: severe, complete interruption of structural
           integrity

Higher grade sprains are associated with increased pain, swelling, and bruising. Treatment may range from a simple compression bandage to an air stirrup and crutches to a cast boot. Undertreatment of ankle sprains may result in chronic weakness and instability. Rupture of the Achilles tendon occurs more frequently in over-forty athletes in general and is often associated with dynamic sports such as basketball and tennis. It usually requires surgical repair.

Fractures of the distal fibula respond to immobilization in a cast boot. More severe fractures of the ankle require the attention of an orthopedic surgeon.

The Leg

Shin splints are painful inflammations of tendinous attachments to the tibia and the periosteum (the connective tissue that covers the bone). They tend to develop gradually and cause pain, aching, and tender areas over the bone. Treatment consists of rest, ice massages, anti-inflammatories, and improved footwear. Stress fractures of the tibia are treated with greater immobilization.

Strains and tears in the muscles of the calf may result from minimal trauma. Often a person will have exercised and rested, then on resumption of activity (sometimes nothing more vigorous than taking a step) experienced a "pop" followed by pain in the calf muscles. Depending on the degree of injury, there may be severe pain, swelling, and bruising. The treatment is ice, elevation, crutches, and extended rest.

The Knee

Common injuries include strains and tears of ligaments, hamstring tendons, and cartilage. These injuries result from sudden twisting motions, hyperextension, or sudden deceleration of the knee joint more than collisions or falls. Pain, joint instability and weakness, effusions (increased fluid in the knee), and a "catching" or "locking" sensation may be noticed. Treatment of these injuries requires an accurate diagnosis and, frequently, the involvement of an orthopedic surgeon.

Injuries involving the kneecap (chondromalacia, subluxation, and idiopathic anterior knee pain) occur more often in women. In contrast to other conditions, such conditions seem to decrease in frequency with advancing age—one thing we can look forward to! They will normally respond to rest, medication, bracing, and strengthening exercises.

The Spine

While contact sports such as football are obvious causes of back injury, so are sports like running, tennis, cycling, weightlifting, and golf. These are mainly muscular and ligamentous injuries, although disk herniations should be considered when pain is more severe, radiates to the extremities, or is associated with numbness, weakness, or bladder or bowel dysfunction.

The Hand and Wrist

Overuse injuries in this area frequently result in tendinitis of the wrist or the thumb extensors (De Quervain's tendinitis). Compressive neuropathy (carpal tunnel syndrome) is less common in sports than in the workplace. These conditions usually respond to rest, medication, and splinting, but they may require referral to a physical therapist or orthopedic specialist.

Fractures, dislocations, and lacerations are common following falls, and range from minor injuries to those requiring surgical repair. Jamming injuries to the fingers can cause disruption of tendon insertions. These require splinting and occasionally surgery.

The Elbow

Soft-tissue inflammation (lateral epicondylitis or tennis elbow, and medial epicondylitis or Little Leaguer's elbow) are the most common conditions and generally respond to rest, ice, and anti-inflammatory medications. Corticosteroid injection and surgical intervention are possible in more severe cases.

Breaks of the radius (one of the two forearm bones) in the elbow area respond to slinging, followed by prompt return to motion. More severe fractures and dislocations require orthopedic intervention.

The Shoulder

Acute injuries include acromioclavicular strains and separations, dislocations, and fractures of the proximal humerus. Strains and tears of the rotator cuff can result both from acute trauma and chronic degeneration. Inflammation of fluid-filled sacs (bursas) causes the pain of bursitis.

The Head

Head injuries are most likely to result from blows (basketball) or falls (cycling). Examination of any head injury resulting in loss of consciousness is mandatory to detect signs of significant brain injury. Headache, dizziness, nausea, forgetfulness, and confusion may reflect a concussion. Exertional headaches can occur in dynamic sports (soccer, football) and weightlifting and are treated with anti-inflammatories.

The Face

Facial injuries include nasal fractures, lacerations, dental injuries, and eye trauma.

Know the Cure

It is commonly assumed that older athletes take longer to heal than their younger competitors do. This is only partially true. Age alone doesn't lengthen the healing process, but the presence of degenerative changes (symptomatic or not) will adversely affect the outcome. Injuries should thus be treated early and aggressively to prevent degenerative changes from occurring and to ensure a speedy return to activity. The treatment, however, will to some extent depend upon the athlete's activity level. Higher-performance athletes may require more aggressive treatment than a casual athlete to whom the injury is less significant.

Delays in treatment do occur. One reason is that an injury may be wrongly ascribed to arthritis or to degeneration. Or the athlete may wish to continue the activity, despite the risk of worsening the injury.

Perhaps the most common error made in acute treatment is that of undertreatment. The adage "better safe than sorry" certainly applies to sports injuries. It's easy, for example, to turn a minor Grade I sprain into a higher grade by not recognizing the potential for worsening. While we all experience the occasional twinge that we can work off, continuing to play with an injury is simply asking for trouble.

There are no clear guidelines to follow for when a physician should be consulted. An obvious deformity requires immediate evaluation, as do the presence of significant bruising, swelling, pain, or limitation of movement. Symptoms that do not resolve in a few days require evaluation.

Know How to Respond

Initial treatment of an acute injury is designed to reduce tissue inflammation, decrease pain, and protect the injured part from further damage. Treatment over the first twenty-four to forty-eight hours is based on the acronym RICE: Rest, Ice, Compression, and Elevation.

Mild analgesics such as acetaminophen, ibuprofen, or naproxen are useful. Stabilization of an injured joint to prevent exacerbation of injury is crucial and can involve use of taping, compression bandage, splints, or crutches.

Overuse injuries may be treated in much the same way, by taking a break from the offending activity, using anti-inflammatories and protective bracing, then progressive mobilization as pain decreases. (With the use of anti-inflammatories, pain relief will come relatively quickly, but the anti-inflammatory effect may take a week or more.) Once pain and inflammation are controlled, treatment can progress to rehabilitation. This phase may involve consultation with a physical therapist or sports medicine therapist to monitor stretching and exercise regimens, measure progress, and possibly employ physical therapies.

The next phase emphasizes the necessity for activity (to prevent muscle wasting) as well as a gradual progression toward full activity. The primary sport may need to be modified in technique, intensity, and frequency. A cross-training program that uses the same muscle groups in a different manner from the primary sport may be employed. Flexibility and stretching exercises restore suppleness to injured tissues while strengthening exercises help prevent reinjury.

The third phase involves return to play. In general, the criteria for resumption of sport are no pain, no swelling, full range of motion, and adequate strength. Failure to pursue rehabilitation to full healing results in a high reinjury rate.

As a last resort for recalcitrant, nonhealing injury, the athlete may need to take up a different sport all together.

Body *and* Spirit

Although this chapter has focused on the body, don't forget that both body and spirit are involved. Medical missionary Dr. John Wilkinson writes, "If the desire for well-being is confined to the body then the result is likely to be not health, but ill-health resulting from a 'healthism' in which the health of the body is regarded as a desirable end in itself. On the other hand, if the desire is confined to the soul or spirit this too will lead to ill-health from neglect of the body."[9]

Yes, Paul focused on spiritual fitness. "Every athlete exercises self-control in all things. They do it to receive a perishable wreath, but we an imperishable. Well, I do not run aimlessly, I do not box as one beating the air; but I pommel my body and subdue it" (1 Corinthians 9:25-27, RSV). Paul may not have been in quest of the fading garland of athletic prowess, but maybe he knew more about this fitness business than we give him credit for. He might even have approved of ten commandments for fitness:

TEN COMMANDMENTS FOR FITNESS

1. Recognize the limitations of your body. It isn't as young as it used to be.
2. Know your goals. Set reasonable, reachable goals for your exercise program.
3. Know your body in detail. Treat it well, with proper nutrition and exercise.
4. Know your sport—its requirements, risks, benefits, preparatory training, and protective measures.
5. Prepare. Start easily and build into activity. Warm up and cool down. Stretch out. Cross-train.
6. Know the most common injuries and the signs of over-training.
7. Know the cure.
8. Don't ignore injury and don't try to be your own doctor. Remember that rehabilitation can prevent reinjury.
9. Seek out expert advice from your physician, a trainer, a sports-medicine practitioner, a professional in your sport, or an organization dedicated to your sport.
10. Have fun. Relax. Enjoy. That's what it's all about.

(The author thanks Connie Younkin and Sara Morris of the Deaconess Billings Clinic library for their assistance in conducting the research for this chapter. Thanks to Barbara Curry, M.D., and Kathy Tyers for reviewing and commenting on the text. Special thanks to Daniel Gall, M.D., and Tim Sanders, Orthopedic PAC.)

SEVEN

Cross-Training: The Key to Fitness After Forty

DON OTIS

Cross-training is the key to staying fit and healthy as our bodies age. "Everything in moderation" is not only a good motto for my diet, but for my exercise too.

—JACQUELINE HANSEN, 52, FORMER WORLD
RECORDHOLDER IN THE MARATHON

Humans are creatures of habit. We like our routines. And the older we get, the more we to tend to resist change. Still, small adjustments in your exercise or routine activities will help you maintain your fitness level and, as we will discover, improve it without adding additional time. Sound too good to be true? It isn't. We all reach a point with repetitive activities when we get bored, stale, discouraged, or undermotivated. There are days that are too dark, humid, gloomy, rainy, or snowy. Or our joints ache. Tiredness reigns. The easy chair beckons. Do any of these descriptions sound familiar? They do for me.

A major theme of this book is that a healthy lifestyle means doing the right things consistently. Yet repetition can lead to overuse as well as boredom. Our aging muscles and joints require alternating amounts of rest and use. How can we accomplish this fine balance? The simplest way is through cross-training. Although injuries aren't the only reason to cross-train, they can provide the impetus we need to try something different. This chapter is designed to help you think about ways to diversify your activities so you will continue to stay active and injury-free well into retirement.

What Is Cross-Training?

Cross-training, or multitasking, simply means choosing a different activity and alternating it with your normal exercise. If your main exercise is running or walking, cross-training activities might include soccer, cycling, swimming (or aquarunning), stairstepping, snowshoeing or Nordic skiing, handball, racquetball, or squash. Perhaps you are thinking, "I can't spend any more time than I already am!" That's okay. Cross-training is not about adding more sports or exercises to your workout schedule. Cross-training is about *substituting* one of the activities mentioned above for what you normally do. While some activities may take more time than others, the point isn't to add more time but to add variety to your workout.

Does Cross-Training Improve Performance?

Cross-training should become an important part of achieving your fitness goals. People stuck in an exercise rut often face a phenomenon known as leveling. We reach a peak in our performance and then level off, getting discouraged because we see little or no ongoing improvement.

Perhaps you are going through the motions (i.e., walking most days) and have become comfortable in your routine. This is fine, unless you want to go faster or farther. One way to do this is to increase the intensity. If you are a walker, include several one- or two-minute jogs each time you are out for your walk. If you are a runner, try doing the same thing by including speed play, adding brief speed segments to your run. For example, on the road you might pick up your pace from one telephone pole to the next (or use some other landmark or increment of time). This increases intensity, builds confidence and speed, and improves the overall benefits (like calorie burning) that you receive from your workout. It also makes the time go by faster and helps build mental toughness.

Or perhaps you have already pushed yourself about as hard as you can. Frankly, most of us have no idea what our physical limitations are because we rarely push ourselves beyond a certain level of discomfort. Susan, a woman in her midforties who is new to exercise, recently told me she found that if she pushed through her initial level of discomfort during exercise, it actually became easier. This doesn't happen all the time, but when it does, it can be an exhilarating feeling. As Michael, a fifty-two-year-old master swimmer explains, "You can't have a great day every day out. But you must get out of your comfort zone a bit." This is true even for the recreational athlete.

The Benefits of Cross-Training

Let's explore some of the benefits of cross-training.

KEEP FIT EVEN WHEN INJURED

Not long ago I suffered a court-related injury to my lateral collateral ligament. This forced me to drastically revise my aerobic workouts to swimming and cycling with one leg. If you do get injured, don't reinjure yourself or delay healing by trying to continue your regular exercise routine. Instead, try cross-training.

Cross-training not only provides an alternative when we're injured, it also helps prevent injuries from occurring in the first place. It reduces the risk of injury because the same muscles, joints, and bones are not subjected to the stresses of repetition when we engage in a variety of sports or activities.

GAIN TOTAL BODY FITNESS

Walking or running does not work the upper-body muscles. Activities such as swimming or weight training do. By including an upper-body workout, you also tone the muscles. By substituting a day or two of swimming or weight training each week, you get a more complete workout.

Strength training helps increase muscle mass and helps prevent osteoporosis, a problem many of us face as we age. It doesn't matter how old you are; you don't have to "get in shape" before starting a strength training regimen. As we age, strength training enables us to continue doing things like moving furniture or yard work, activities that can be difficult for those whose muscles have begun to atrophy due to disuse.

In her fitness column, Kathy Smith says, "A lot of women think that their strength-training regimens must differ from a man's. Not true. Males and females both have...the same number of bones and the same number of muscles and they all work on the same principles."[1] The heavier weights I used to lift in my twenties and thirties have given way to lighter weights and additional repetitions. As we get older, heavier weights can put additional stress on shoulders and joints. If you are just getting started, lift lighter weights—though choose weights that are heavy enough to provide adequate resistance.

If you have never lifted weights before but want to begin, educate yourself about muscle groups and resistance training. Go to a local gym, YMCA, or hire a personal trainer (at least for a few months). Proper instruction in the beginning will help you avoid injury and maximize the benefits of your weight-training program. You will also learn specific exercises for toning weak muscle groups. Once you know what you're doing, you can buy your own weights and keep them at home. If you plan to stay active at a gym, learn how to use weight machines as well as free weights. Though most of us cannot afford the expensive machines found at most gyms, you can still work out at home with free weights or cheaper weight machines found at many athletic chain stores.

REDUCE EXERCISE BOREDOM

Common sense tells us that variety eliminates monotony. It helps sustain long-term interest in fitness and exercise. During the winter months, I do most of my running indoors. This doesn't mean, however, that all I use is a treadmill. To be honest, I get tired of the jogging machines. Most of my indoor work includes a combination of treadmill, elliptical trainer, StairMaster, and stationary bike. By moving from one machine to the next, I rarely get bored. But even when I run on a treadmill, I don't just set the speed and plod through my run. Instead, I often will run quarter-mile intervals at a faster pace. Other people like to use the incline feature, which simulates hiking, walking, or running uphill.

If you adopt a new sport or begin cross-training, don't expect that your present conditioning will automatically carry you through. No matter how "in shape" you are, moving from walking or running to a court sport or weight training will involve new muscles. That is also the case when moving between seasonal sports over the course of a year. When you begin a new activity, take it slow, and let the new muscle groups adapt to the unfamiliar motion and new stress.

IMPROVE YOUR PERFORMANCE

You can maintain or increase your stamina if your cross-training activities include an aerobic workout. You will build the heart muscle, which in turn increases blood volume and flow. As muscles receive more oxygen, they work harder and longer without fatigue.

A runner whose legs are tired from overexertion one day can switch to cycling or swimming the next and get an excellent workout that will improve his overall performance in his primary sport. Again, when you swim or run, your lung capacity often increases dramatically. You will experience less fatigue and be able to push yourself even harder. Intensity, as we mentioned earlier, is a primary ingredient in improving your times and performances.

But the performance benefits are not only physical. Cross-training helps build a mental edge. The more you mix up aerobic activities, the more you and your body know what it feels like to physically push yourself. God has made your body and mine with the unique ability to remember or recall previous conditions. If you have been exercising for a while, perhaps you can recall how sore you were when you started. Chances are, you don't feel as sore when you exercise now as you did when you first began. (And if you are just getting started, the good news is that your muscles will get used to the work load.)

BURN MORE CALORIES

One of the benefits of cross-training is that we burn more calories. Think of your body as an engine. To keep it running you need to provide good fuel (something other than doughnuts!). To lose weight, you have to either burn up more fuel or reduce the amount of fuel you put in your engine. The best kind of weight loss comes through a two-pronged approach of burning calories and reducing or altering intake (for example, choosing high-fiber foods over sugary snacks). The more calories you burn, the more fat you will lose. As you lose weight, you will discover greater efficiency and stamina. The fat you lose through cross-training will also make a difference in your overall performance in other sports or activities.

CULTIVATE COORDINATION

Linear activities such as walking, running, swimming, and cycling provide some of the very best aerobic conditioning opportunities. Cross-training, however, makes it possible to supplement these linear exercises with sports or activities that require lateral movements. These can improve your reflex time and overall coordination. Lateral activities include tennis, handball, racquetball, basketball, and aerobics classes.

God made us with ankle, knee, and hip joints that are effective in forward and reverse. Quick side-to-side motion, however, places extra stress on our ligaments and connective tissues. As a result, there are scores of middle-aged men and women who have damaged their legs playing basketball, street hockey, court sports, or skiing. While these activities can provide an excellent workout, they also elevate our risk of injury.

For those of us over forty, sports that require quick lateral movement should be started slowly and then only after adequate warmup. Aaron Branigan, one of the top racquetball players in the world, told me he spends no less than thirty minutes to one hour stretching and warming up before playing a high-intensity game. If this is true for one of the best players in the world, it is even more important for those of us who are older.

Alternating Activities: Case Studies in Cross-Training

A little more than ten years ago, I prepared for Ventura's Gold Coast Triathlon with its fifteen-hundred-meter open-ocean swim. The course turned out to be seventeen hundred meters in cool, cloudy conditions with choppy waves. Seaweed kept getting caught on my arms as I took stroke after miserable stroke. It wasn't much fun. In fact, by the time I reached the beach, I was hypothermic. My feet were numb. As I exited the water and was running up the beach, I heard a crack. My toe was broken. I completed the race in a shoe soaked with blood from the break.

It had become too painful to continue my run training with a broken toe, yet I still planned to compete in another race a month away. So instead of abandoning my plans altogether, I improvised. I kept swimming and cycling, but I wasn't sure what to do about the running part. At the gym I started using a versa climber—a cheap but effective stationary device that simulates climbing. There was virtually no impact, which allowed me to continue my aerobic training.

Let's look at some of the alternating activities others use to keep active and fit.

- Michael is a fifty-two-year-old accountant. In college and afterward, he was an excellent runner. More than a decade ago, he realized that high-intensity, competitive running could eventually damage his knees and joints. So he took up swimming again and has become one of the fastest in the world in his age group. Michael's decision to move from a higher-impact to a lower-impact sport has proven a smart one. Though he does weight training twice a week to supplement his swimming, he spends most of his time in the pool.

- Loni is a forty-year-old administrator who recently started going to the gym. She began by doing water aerobics and graduated to a regular aerobics class. Today she walks or jogs for forty-five minutes or uses a stationary bike. She also lifts weights, something she says she was afraid to do a couple of years ago.

- Bill is an eighty-year-old semiretired minister who started exercising just before his sixtieth birthday. He is careful about what he eats, maintains his weight, and walks almost every day. Bill uses a stationary cycle and occasionally lifts weights to stay toned. He encourages people who are older not to become a slave to exercise but to "get up and get going." He says, "Do what you can, but don't make it so hard that you want to quit."

- Jim is a fifty-six-year-old former university professor. He rides his bicycle whenever he can, pans for gold, hikes, plays an excellent game of squash, and lifts weights. Jim is in great shape and maintains perfect weight. I have seen him outplay other squash players in their twenties. Jim's balanced approach to exercise includes making it fun so he can continue for many years to come.

• Randy is a fifty-year-old radio program host at a Christian radio station in Texas. He never liked to exercise when he was young. He got started a few years ago by accident when he received a temporary membership to a local gym as a station promotion. Today Randy says he is stronger than at any other time in his life because he has been in regular weight training. Randy says learning to say no to yourself in the physical arena leads to self-discipline in the spiritual arena. He balances his weight training by getting up very early several days a week to run.

While the benefits of cross-training can add variety and enjoyment to your exercise routine, some of us are not content with just staying in shape. For those who want to compete in a road race or set personal goals, the next chapter will provide help in taking your training to the next level.

EIGHT

Training for Athletic Success

JEFF MITCHUM

*We are conditioned to think that great athletes should stop competing
when they're no longer great. But if you enjoy running as much as I do,
what's wrong with continuing to do it even if you are no longer one
of the best?*

—STEVE SCOTT, AMERICAN RECORDHOLDER IN THE MILE

For most of us, there comes a time in our lives when we want
to break out of the routine. We want to test our limits. We want to
know how fast or how far we can go. That's what this chapter is
about. If you are one of those people who is bored with the same
fitness pattern, this chapter will add new life to your program. It
will give you a jump-start to run that road race, enter a master's
swim meet, or simply prepare for a long ride or hike. While not all
of us have competitive instincts, some of us do. By the time we
turn forty, fifty, or sixty, some of us want to know how we measure
up to other people our age. Thankfully, most races have age-group
categories—recognizing that those of us over forty are rarely going
to beat athletes in their twenties. As we get older, however, most

of us are competing against ourselves (which is as it should be). Natalie, a forty-something housewife and businesswoman, is a good example of someone who is motivated by goal setting.

Five years ago Natalie was 303 pounds. She was depressed, out-of-breath, and had difficulty walking. It was a visit to her doctor that shook Natalie up. In no uncertain terms he told her, "Lose weight or die." She was too young to accept the inevitability of an early death, so she took matters into her own hands. It wasn't easy. Today she says it was the power of the Holy Spirit that helped her make the slow, necessary changes. Natalie began by walking and soon lost ten pounds. Then she attended Weight Watchers where she found accountability and support. Although she was apprehensive about it, she joined a health club and started attending aerobics classes. (She stayed in the back of the class.) Her weight kept coming down.

Then one day an acquaintance suggested she consider entering an open-lake swim. Natalie was hooked on the idea. The goal seemed impossible, but she worked hard and eventually completed a nearly two-mile lake swim! Now she needed another goal, so she entered a five-kilometer race (3.1 miles) and finished it. Not long afterward she set her sights on an even loftier goal—a marathon. She found a training partner, solicited guidance from an experienced runner, then started training for the Portland Marathon. Again she overcame the odds and finished the race. Today Natalie teaches an aerobics class. She says it is an enormous relief to know that she is going to live. She believes the weight loss combined with the athletic goals have enabled her to encourage people, help women build self-esteem, and become a better businesswoman.

As anyone who has tried to tame and bridle their body for better performance knows, there are days when defeat knocks at the door. The single greatest stress and challenge I have ever put my flesh through was during the Ironman Triathlon in Hawaii. The evening before the race I unwisely broke with prerace protocol and ate a spicy meal in Kona. The following day's race was miserable. My mistake was simple: I broke with my normal race plan and paid an enormous price. I have learned, often the hard way, that athletic success is found in the small choices we make.

The Key to Improvement

Serious athletes are familiar with the term *periodization training* or *cycle training*. This is a method used by every Olympic medalist and by coaches throughout the world. Periodization training is an exercise plan to build your fitness level by alternating appropriate amounts of rest and work over four-week cycles.

As Christians we understand that the Bible is the solid foundation that gives us direction to live the way He has designed us. It is a starting point for success, a building block for our future triumphs. Similarly, in athletics, periodization training is a plan or basis for our own physical and competitive improvement. Without it, your performances will not significantly improve.

Periodization consists of three distinct phases, each with a special target in mind.

PHASE ONE

The first phase is a lower heart rate and "long slow distance" (better known in the fitness world as LSD). You may spend between one and three months in this phase, depending on your present level of conditioning. It is the base you need for success in the next two phases.

The goal is to develop an aerobic base. Consequently you are also developing your slow-twitch muscles by keeping your heart rate down with longer sustained efforts. These are muscle fibers that have a slower contraction time. What does this mean to you? These muscles use oxygen for power and provide the endurance necessary for maintaining long physical efforts. They are found mostly in the legs, hips, thighs, trunk, and back. Muscles change and develop with regular exercise, but the effects differ, depending on whether you engage in strength, speed, or endurance training.

Your focus on this initial training phase should last about three months. This phase helps to prepare your body for the endurance workload or sustained effort without risking injury by doing up-tempo workouts. The off-season and winter months are an ideal time to concentrate on this initial phase. Each week, include one sustained effort lasting forty to sixty minutes.

For example, if you are planning to run a ten-kilometer race (6.2 miles), the sixty minutes of slow jogging will prepare your slow-twitch muscles for the longer effort. Of course, running isn't the only sport or activity that those of us over forty set our sights on. There are countless athletes over forty who compete in triathlons (swim-bike-run), biathlons (generally a run-bike-run), master's swimming, and backpacking or climbing. The idea in this first phase is not speed. It is to prepare your muscles to handle the stamina required to complete an activity without injury.

The majority of people over forty who set their sights on a tangible athletic goal choose running. If you have never competed in a race before, I suggest you start out by simply trying to finish your first race without walking—don't worry about the speed. If you have done some aerobic exercise on a regular basis (three or more times each week), you will find it easier to achieve your goal. As a case in point, let's say you want to run a ten-kilometer race. Begin by selecting a race that is no less than eight to twelve weeks away. If you can already jog ten minutes, your first week of training should include at least one longer run—say fifteen minutes or more. Run it at a comfortable pace. The objective is to add at least five or six minutes a week to your longest run. By the time you toe the starting line, remember to go out slowly—slower than you think you can run. It is better to finish strong than to start fast and burn out at the end. Most newer runners over forty achieve their goal and then wonder what to do next. There is an inevitable prerace exhilaration and then letdown afterward. If you enjoyed the racing experience, make plans for another race or establish new goals. It may be a longer race, a more difficult run, or a faster time.

After you complete the first phase, you are ready to increase the tempo of your workouts.

PHASE TWO

This second phase of your training is a combination of quantity (usually measured in time or distance) and quality (usually measured in increased effort). The emphasis is on acquiring added strength and improving or maintaining your aerobic fitness level, which comes from a combination of longer sustained efforts coupled with quality work. In other words, the intensity of your efforts increases.

Using the example I just mentioned, if you only want to complete a race and don't really want to improve your times, you can skip phases two and three. If, however, you want to improve your strength and speed, these last two phases are essential. Strength and what is called "burst training" cause muscle fibers to enlarge, increasing in diameter. This is why sprinters are built like body-builders and distance runners are thin. As we get older, muscle mass is important to our performance. This second phase, this building of strength, is important to your performance success, but it also helps you avoid injury. Muscle strength can be developed in a variety of ways, but resistance training (like weight training) is one of the best. If you are a jogger or runner trying to strengthen your leg muscles for that ten-kilometer race, cycling (stationary or on the road) is also excellent.

These increasingly intense efforts of phase two should not be beyond your anaerobic threshold. *Anaerobic* means "without oxygen." We have all seen people who were out of shape and gasping for breath following an intense physical effort. It is most often the result of a buildup of lactic acid, which puts your muscles into "oxygen debt." We see this in the final meters of middle-distance races where runners seem to be pushing hard but the muscles struggle to respond. This is not what you are after.

This second training phase has been enormously valuable to my own racing seasons. I am not gifted with good, natural strength. So to compensate I do strength training—squats, lunges, and calf raises. This has enabled me to improve my strength and achieve better performances.

If you make it successfully through the first two phases, you are ready for the final training phase. But before you make this transition, let me implore you, as a pastor and a trainer, to be honest with yourself about your abilities. The worst thing you can do is try to do too much too soon. By overtraining, you can actually weaken your performance, risk injury, and get discouraged. At some time or another, many of us are tempted to do someone else's workout, allowing ourselves to get pulled into another person's fitness regimen. If you yield to that temptation, though, there is the danger that you will not do what you should do or that you will overdo what you shouldn't. By trying to train at an inappropriate level, you also risk the possibility of an unproductive workout.

Phase Three

The single greatest mistake in training is doing the same workout, the same way, at the same heart rate. Such workouts are neither hot nor cold but lukewarm. You will become stale doing this. Instead, you need to shift gears—increase the tempo. As earlier chapters have already discussed, cross-training can help older competitive athletes build aerobic capacity (endurance) and avoid injury. The focus of this last stage is on improving your speed—and consequently your racing times.

Using a ten-kilometer race as an example again, you build speed work into your weekly mileage. This doesn't mean you stop your long runs each week. Depending on your age and commitment, intervals can be run at a nearby running track, park, or even the roads. (I recommend a running track so you can measure your progress.) A series of quarter miles or half-miles slightly faster than your anticipated race pace build mental tenacity, leg speed, and strength. Give yourself between two and three minutes rest between each interval. For example, you would run eight to ten times around a quarter-mile track (or the equivalent), or you would run eight hundred meters, which is two laps around a running track, six to eight times. Mile repeats, run at race pace or faster, can be substituted for the shorter intervals.

Don't try to fast-forward to phase three. Instead, use the earlier two training phases to lose weight and train your cardiovascular system. Use phase three to train your fast-twitch muscles. The purpose of these muscles is to provide rapid responses and quick shifts in direction. These muscles furnish both strength and speed (used in basketball, fast running, tennis, and other court sports).

If there is a picture of what this third phase is all about, it would be an Indy 500 formula car—fast, but with endurance. The purpose of phase three is to develop speed, quality, and strength. During my training and racing, I often wonder, "How can I go so long and do it fast?" It comes by doing high-tempo workouts. This is not to say that you won't get strong doing a lot of exercises (volume) or by focusing on quality work. However, to go over the edge and reach an elite level you must do both. Like a bow and the strings of a violin, both elements need to come together to make beautiful sounds.

To accomplish phase three, your volume needs to decrease as your intensity increases. This is a basic formula for all endurance athletes; quality should begin to replace quantity in the final phase of periodization training. Make sure you are pushing yourself at least one or two times a week at about 85 percent of your maximum capability (you can find the formula for this in chapter 3). Be sure to schedule adequate recovery time of at least twenty-four to thirty-six hours between these intense sessions. In this third phase, work to find a balance between sustained, hard efforts and adequate recovery time. Recovery is an important ingredient in the entire training process.

Overtraining: How to Avoid
the Temptation

If you use periodization training, you are disciplined in the subtle balance between proper training, rest, and intense physical exercise. Remember, when you overtrain you risk injury. Injuries are a reminder that you did not listen to the still, small voice in your overall training regimen. If you don't make time for rest, your day of judgment will eventually arrive. General fatigue, decreased libido, pulled muscles, and sore knees, ankles, and hip joints are just the tip of the iceberg for those who refuse to pace themselves.

A habitually overtrained friend of mine is a classic example. "Bob" is a likable guy who is also extremely motivated in his training. In fact, Bob is a bit obsessive. He believes, as many athletes do, that more is always better. If he is supposed to run easy one day, he can be effortlessly swayed to change his schedule. If someone invites him to go on and do a track workout, too, Bob's going to ignore his recovery phase and do the hard workout anyway. His reason? He says, "There's always time to rest tomorrow."

One day my training partner and I were scheduled to do a hard 120-mile bike ride on the "doughnut bike loop" (Dudley's Bakery is the place for carbo-loading) through Santa Isabel and Mount Palomar near my home in the San Diego area. It was sure to be one of those great bonding experiences that ends in physical exhaustion (better known as "melting"). Guess who shows up on his "easy day" to ride along with us? You guessed it. For Bob, breaking rocks on a prison chain gang would be a vacation! I asked him, "Aren't you supposed to ride easy today?" "Yeah," he told me, "but I can ride easy tomorrow."

Are you overdoing it? Let's take a look at some of the telltale signs:

- edginess
- insomnia
- depression
- loss of appetite or weight
- chronic illness
- heart rate is five to ten beats-per-minute higher in the morning
- inability to raise your heart rate
- family or marriage problems
- decreased libido
- night sweats
- lack of interest in Bible study, prayer, fellowship, and worship
- refusing to consider the possibility that you are overtraining (denial)
- obsessive devotion to your exercise regimen

As you can see, overtraining and underresting create real problems—both physical and otherwise. An excess of anything, even fitness and training, is tantamount to idolatry. Forty-three-year-old Ruth Wysocki, a member of the 1984 U.S. Olympic team, makes this observation about her training: "I try to keep my life in balance and not let any one thing become too dominant. I believe that anyone can make the time for working out and staying fit; it's just a matter of how important it is to you."[1] In this brief statement, Wysocki wisely synthesizes the necessity of staying fit with the equally important need to keep our lives in perspective.

To put it bluntly, if you are overtraining, you are not living your life as God intended. We call it overtraining, but it is really disobedience. If your lifestyle includes obsessive training, you need to ask (and honestly answer) the question, "Have I gone too far?" We must allow God to speak to our hearts, and then we must be willing to follow His direction. If you are literally running after the wrong things and you are not spending time in reading the Bible, prayer, fellowship, and worship, your life is not in balance.

The Right Training Partner

Jesus must have had a good reason for sending His disciples out two by two. He must have understood something about the power of companionship. I know firsthand that working out with a partner can be beneficial to our motivation and overall improvement.

A woman named Sara is one of the best training partners I ever had. She had a strong training ethic and a wonderful mental disposition. Even though she was a tough competitor, she didn't have the ego to go along with it. She also had terrific athletic talent, yet she never tried to prove how fast she was. This is the kind of person you want as a training partner—not some egomaniac who is always trying to prove his or her worthiness to you. What is the point of having a training partner if all he or she wants to do is beat you up every hill?

When lining up your own training partner, look for a person with a similar fitness level and goals. Unfortunately, it can be difficult to find someone with compatible skills and interests. For example, it isn't unusual for someone at church to ask to bike or run with me. While I appreciate the offer and the company, my concern is what I should do if he is unable to keep up. Rather than planning to leave him in my dust, if I need to run, I tell him to bring his mountain bike and we can talk and train at the same time. If he wants to ride his bike with me, I ask him to leave his bike at home and to borrow my Honda Elite 150 instead.

Another quality to look for in a training partner is dependability. I had one partner who was consistently a half-hour late at our meeting points. Finally the day came to share the truth in love. I smiled when I told him that God required me to use my time wisely and that by waiting for him all the time I was not doing that! I was pleasantly surprised by his response, and he became one of the best partners I have had.

When choosing a training partner, find someone with a similar focus in life. Since training is a subtle mix of mind, body, and spirit, what affects me physically also affects me emotionally. And what affects me emotionally can affect me spiritually. Several years ago I had a partner I did light training with. It became apparent that he was more interested in chasing other women than he was in investing in his own marriage. He would say, "Look at her!" when he saw a woman he thought was attractive. I asked him not to do this. As a Christian, I didn't want to subject myself to any more of the world's temptations than I was already bombarded with. Don't settle for someone whose values are so different that all you have in common is training the physical person.

Remember the wonderful benefits of finding the right training partner. It helps your workout go by faster, and it is a good distraction. You know the old adage "Misery loves company." This is no less true for training.

Final Words About Serious Training

Since wisdom is the right application of knowledge—or knowing what to do with the information we do have—don't get caught up in all the latest training fads. There are a growing number of fads in the marketplace today that all say they can make you a better athlete. Be careful. Look at the empirical (researched) or anecdotal (hearsay) evidence. I have seen athletes throw caution to the wind and try supplements that were nothing more than steroids.

A few years ago I called the advertising manager at a popular multisport magazine to ask if he knew one of their ads was for a "nutritional supplement" that was actually a steroid. An athlete who took this supplement could test positive for a banned substance. The ad manager told me he would "look into it," but the ads ran for another six months. Not long afterward several top-level professional athletes who were using the advertised supplement actually did test positive for a banned substance and were suspended. Such situations can be avoided by investigating solid, long-term studies and knowing what your body needs. Knowing the Lord, having a basic understanding of nutrition, proper training, adequate rest, and recovery are the cornerstones to making significant athletic improvements—not quick-fix supplements or the latest herbal energy mixes.

The advantages to physical activity and a regular fitness routine are just part of maintaining an overall healthy lifestyle. Even the most vigorous exercise will not counteract an unhealthy diet. To live physically healthy, we need to integrate the other part of our physical bodies: what we put into them. While there are innumerable fad diets and quick-fix solutions for losing weight fast or bulking up, the next chapter will concentrate on some spiritual dimensions to healthful eating and healthy living.

NINE

Eating Right for Healthy Living

MARY RUTH SWOPE, PH.D.

Our goal is to make sure that we take into our bodies all that we need to maintain excellent health and eliminate those things from our diet that we know damage our health.

—JUDY LINDBERG MCFARLAND

By the seventh grade, most Americans have learned the basic rules of healthful living. They are simple, inexpensive, easy to do. Almost changeless in concept. So what's the problem? Why aren't more of us actually living our lives in a healthy way? The problem is we resist the rules' reality. We want "more for less." Or we desire something new and more exciting, something quick and effortless. Or we believe that the miracle cure for healthy living is just waiting to be concocted in a scientific laboratory by highly educated professionals.

Americans today—young and old alike—are struggling with obesity and the diseases that accompany it. Being unfit is now the norm. Forty million adult Americans (about 20 percent of the population) are overweight. Obesity is increasing in all major races and among men and women alike. It is America's number-one malnutrition problem and a serious risk factor that we cannot ignore. Yet it is one thing most of us can do something about—by eating healthfully, exercising, and controlling our food intake. By doing so, we can control hypertension, diabetes, certain kinds of cancer, cardiovascular disease, endocrine abnormalities, pulmonary problems, certain types of arthritis, and even some psychological disorders.[1]

If we want to be healthy and disease-free, we must study and apply the scientifically proven, time-honored principles of health. There is no other way to achieve a constant state of wellness. There are no shortcuts.

The Search for Proper Balance

All living, rejuvenating, healing processes are intimately related to four key ingredients: the work of nutrients, the consumption of adequate amounts of pure water, the absence of high levels of toxins achieved through simple exercise, and adequate amounts of rest and sleep in a stress-controlled environment. For many of us, one or more of these areas is out of balance.

The whole world has served as a proving ground for our physical condition. What we regularly consume can be a remarkably accurate predictor of our length and quality of life, our reproductive ability, our physical size, vitality, disease patterns, mental acuity, and productivity. All we really need is to eat a selection of foods that supplies appropriate amounts of the essential nutrients and energy. The challenge is to put into practice what we know to be true.

The Food and Drug Administration has defined a drug as any substance that cures, heals, relieves, mitigates, or treats a symptom. Ironically, there is a plethora of medical literature showing that nutrients can better be used as medicines than prescription drugs to correct imbalances at the molecular level, which often leads to reversing illnesses, including chronic degenerative disease. Today, however, few medical professionals have practiced medicine based on a *nutrition as medicine* concept. Nonetheless, it is basic to the understanding of how to change sick cells into healthy cells.

FOOD AS MEDICINE

Hippocrates is known today as the "Father of Medicine." He lived four hundred years before Christ and doctored in his native Greece with such skill that men from all over the ancient world came to learn from him.

Hippocrates is credited as saying, "Food is your best medicine, and the best foods are the best medicines." I have also found this to be true. For me, however, the true genius of Hippocrates lies in the fact that he recognized the necessity of treating illness *consistent with nature*. He believed that the natural forces within our bodies are truly the healers of disease.

Most medical care is based upon treatment modalities that are unnatural. For example, their main tools are drugs, chemotherapy, and surgery—all things that often debilitate patients and leave them with side effects requiring additional doctor visits, surgery, or hospitalization.

The results of this approach are shocking. Iatrogenic disease (disease induced inadvertently by a physician or a prescribed treatment) now ranks as the third cause of death in the United States; only heart disease and cancer are ahead of it. We must educate ourselves regarding the type of medical treatment that best serves our need for solving health problems. Even more important, we must educate ourselves on how to use nutrition as preventive and curative medicine. Cells made strong through good nutrition will build or rebuild an immune system that will resist and reverse the illnesses so prevalent in our society today. (We will explore the natural solutions for producing healthy cells later in this chapter).

Nutrition's Spiritual Dimension

After sixty years of interest, experience, and education in nutrition, I have a clear understanding of God's original design for healthy cells. Let me share what I believe is true based upon the Bible.

If we begin with the biblical account of humanity's origin (we were made by God from the dust of the earth), it is easy to explain the rest. In Genesis 1:11 we read, "Then God said, 'Let the land produce vegetation: seed-bearing plants and trees,'" and in verse 12, "And God saw that it was good."

On the sixth day of Creation, the Bible says that God created man and woman. And God told them, "I give you every seed-bearing plant on the face of the whole earth and every tree that has fruit with seed in it. They will be yours for food" (1:29). Now this is the simple truth: God created a magnificent human body. Psalm 139:14 points out that we are "fearfully and wonderfully made." God then purposefully made every perfect provision through the food supply from the earth for our body's growth, maintenance, and repair of tissue (healing), without any opportunity for a physical or chemical conflict. I believe that scientists will eventually prove that Genesis's "seed-bearing plants and trees"—along with pure air, pure water, enough exercise, and adequate rest (both physical and mental)—are the keys to as perfect health as it is possible to have on this planet.

If cells are given the proper ingredients, in the right amounts, at the right time, in the right cell environment, they will reproduce themselves and live in health without the use of any other outside substance. Nobel Prize–winning scientist Alexis Carrel proved this point by keeping a chicken heart alive in a test tube for years, just by providing it daily with nature's cell recipe (food) and removing the toxins that were given off as it used the nutrients. Cells are capable of living, growing, reproducing, healing themselves, and performing special functions only so long as the blood, muscles, organs, glands, and body fluids bring them the proper concentrations of vitamins, minerals, amino acids, fatty substances, oxygen, glucose, and phytochemicals required by the body's internal environment.

All of the functions of the body depend upon the health of the organs; the health of the organs, in turn, depends on the health of the tissues that compose the organs. The health of the tissues depends on healthy individual cells; the health of the cells depends on the supply of nutrients in the blood. The supply of nutrients in the blood depends on the foods and beverages we consume. Natural foods are best. They are the perfect sources of all the nutrients needed or required for health. Life can come only from life. All-natural foods, as provided in the beginning of time by nature (as God designed it), are the best sources of life. Manufactured food products are always inferior to foods that nature provides.

ADAM AND EVE'S KITCHEN

What was the food preparation like back in the Garden of Eden? In Adam and Eve's kitchen, would we have found a can opener, a microwave oven, a container of MSG, an 18-cubic-foot side-by-side refrigerator, or a set of aluminum cookware? Would they have had a four-burner gas or electric stove or a grill?

In their cupboards would there be cardboard boxes filled with thousands of choices of "stuff to eat" (foodless foods)? How about metal cans? Would they have preservatives, purified salt, pesticides, and countless other things that the body has no "ready recipe" for using very well? Would we have found bags of white sugar, white rice, white flour, white shortening, white salt, or powdered white milk?

In their pantry would there have been carton after carton of bottled beverages—many containing caffeine, phosphoric acid, large amounts of sugar, coloring, and preservatives, which can lead to obesity and put a person at risk for cancer, diabetes, heart disease, osteoporosis, kidney and liver damage, plus a host of other degenerative diseases?

You Are What You Eat

What we eat, drink, and breathe becomes part of the cell structure of our bodies. And the composition of our bodies determines precisely every aspect of our being—the health or sickness of our hair, skin, eyes, glands, nails, teeth, bones, organs, blood, and all other living substances. This is why it is important to have some knowledge about food and its relationship to how you look, feel, and act. It is also why it is important to be wise in applying that knowledge to your everyday life.

Too many of us are not paying attention to the kind of bodies that result from diets filled with pretzels and soda, hamburgers and french fries, candy bars, refined and processed boxed foods, pickles and potato chips, beef steak with mashed potatoes and gravy, hot dogs with white buns, ice cream, bacon and sausage with white toast, biscuits and gravy, doughnuts, croissants and coffee, to name just a few of our popular poor-quality favorites. I would put all of these items on a list of foods to eliminate first. These foods are poor examples of nutrient-dense foods that lead to good cell health. If you want to improve your health, abandoning these foods is a prudent place to begin.

Healthy cells require the right types and the right amounts of six major classes of nutrients: proteins, carbohydrates, fats, vitamins, minerals, and water. Besides these basic nutrients, there are enzymes, neurotransmitters, prostaglandins, auxins, phytochemicals, and probably many others not yet known or understood very well. These substances perform three major functions: building tissue (growth), repairing and maintaining tissue, and supplying energy for all internal and external work.

POPULAR MISPERCEPTIONS ABOUT PROTEIN

Protein foods digest into smaller units called amino acids (there are more than twenty of them), which are the muscle builders. Many Americans wholeheartedly believe that meats (especially steak) are the preferred protein foods for building healthy cells. Only a small minority believe that beans, nuts, grains, seeds, eggs, and milk can build a muscular football player or a boxing champ. Yet research, both ancient and modern, shows that these foods rank nutritionally with animal protein.

Furthermore, Americans by the millions are producing unhealthy cells by eating too much meat. Here are examples of the effects:

- an overproduction of purines in the blood, which results in too much uric acid (This is associated with gout and kidney stones.)
- an overtaxing of the cells, which leads to overworking (and potentially enlarging) the liver
- an overproduction of ammonia, a natural by-product of protein metabolism, which adversely affects the function of RNA and DNA, the genetic blueprint that tells healthy cells how to reproduce
- a shortened life span

These are just a few of the disadvantages of a diet that includes one or two servings of meat every day. A better balance includes two or three servings of meat *per week*. This is adequate for good cell health. It is best to keep total protein calories limited to about 10 to 15 percent of your total calorie intake.

CARBOHYDRATES

Healthy cells also require the right mix and the right amounts of complex and simple carbohydrate foods—the starches and sugars. Complex starches include whole-grain breads, corn, lentils, rice, oatmeal, most beans, spaghetti, noodles, barley, potatoes, and similar foods. Simple carbohydrate foods are all sugars. These foods require almost no digestion; they are quick energy. The best sources of quick energy are, of course, the natural ones—not manufactured sugars. The sugar in fruits, fresh and dried, are less likely to throw the body out of chemical balance—making us tired, nervous, lazy, fuzzy-minded, short-tempered, restless, or apprehensive.

Half of all the foods needed for good health should be from the complex carbohydrate group, with only 10 percent coming from the simple sugar foods. As you plan your diet, be sure to get about 50 percent of your total calories from carbohydrates.

The Facts About Fats

The subject of fats is hotly debated. Are they good for us or not? Some specialists say yes, and others say no. Here are a few facts you can believe.

Fats are absolutely necessary for building and maintaining healthy cells. They are an essential part of the way God made our bodies and are the principal way the body stores energy. Fat performs many good functions, such as making us feel satisfied after a meal and giving us energy. Fats insulate our nerves. They carry certain vitamins. They also act as an insulator against loss of body heat.

Yet fats also can be great offenders to cell health. They can be deposited in cells in forms that cannot be broken down. This is especially true of animal fats—including lard, butter, and saturated fat. A diet that contains a high proportion of saturated fat is one of the factors contributing to heart disease. Some people believe that simply substituting margarine for pure butter will solve their problem with this form of fat. That is not true. The body's cells have no recipe for breaking down the plastic-like substance that results when hydrogen is added to the vegetable oils in making margarine and vegetable shortenings. The cells have no alternative but to lay down the substance on artery walls—hardening and plugging these blood vessels. The best cell health results when the greater proportion of fats eaten are in such foods as avocados, nuts, nut butters of all kinds, sunflower and sesame seeds, firm ripe olives and olive oil, other seed oils, and butter in small quantities (no more than two tablespoons per day).

Americans eat 40 percent of their total calories in the form of fat (through hamburgers, hot dogs, lunch meats, bacon, ham, fried meats, chips of all kinds, doughnuts, and so forth). To prevent diseases directly related to a high fat intake (high blood pressure, heart disease, hardening of the arteries, obesity, clogged colon, liver and kidney diseases), we must lower our fat intake from the present 40 percent to 20 to 25 percent of our total calories. We must cut down on the use of fat, eliminate or reduce the use of oil-based mayonnaise, deep-fried foods, ice cream, sour cream, margarine, pork products, lard, and fatty meats. Replace these with poultry and fish that reduce the intake of saturated fats. Drink low-fat and nonfat milk instead of whole milk. By making a few changes in your diet, you will promote greater cell health.

VITAMINS AND MINERALS

Vitamins and minerals are well known to be regulators of all body processes—both those that build up cells (anabolic) and those that tear down cells (catabolic). These are absolutely necessary for cell health. The prefix *vita* means "life," and cells of every kind need vitamins and minerals in order to sustain life. Natural minerals are put to the most efficient use by the body's cells. Vitamins and minerals in the form of fruits and vegetables are natural, pure, and whole. They never cause stress, adverse side effects, or disease in the cells.

Cells require small amounts of these nutrients. Nutrition companies, catalogs, and advertisements that suggest megadoses of natural nutrients are misleading. Such doses are not necessary. Neither is the use of synthetic products. While toxicity is unlikely if the sources of water-soluble vitamins are natural foods, large doses of vitamin supplements can actually reach toxic levels. It would be almost impossible, however, to have hypervitaminosis (or too many minerals) while eating fresh, natural foods. It is an important basic rule that if you eat a wide variety of foods in all categories, you will be adding to your own high quality of health.

As they do with so many other health-related issues, Americans continue to believe there is a quick solution to their vitamin deficiencies. While the absence of certain vitamins can certainly cause serious problems, their presence does not make up for a deficient diet. The only disease a vitamin will cure is the one caused by a deficiency of that vitamin. Vitamins are not cure-alls for such vague symptoms as tiredness, depression, or anxiety.

There are many good sources that describe the forty-plus nutrients and their function. Look for books on this subject or summary charts within books that will answer more specific questions about vitamins and minerals.

Cell Health Is True Wealth

If all the scientists in the world could agree on a single fact, it would be this: *Life begins, is maintained, and ends at the cellular level.* The health of single cells holds the key to the health of the whole organism. Why is this so? Because single cells of a similar type clump together to form tissues, and tissues cluster to form organs. To keep individual cells healthy is to experience health in the whole body. In reverse, when individual cells become unhealthy, tissues can become unhealthy; if the process is unchecked, disease or death can result.

Cells are the basic units of life. They are ultimately and uniquely responsible for all functions of living matter. Their duties are specific. Yet when they are considered collectively, all the functions of the organism are perfectly met when the cells are healthy. For cells to be healthy, a narrow range of circumstances must be present for them to live and reproduce while they maintain homeostasis (a steady state). Once there is too great a change in the set of conditions required for functioning, cells die and the organism risks losing its equilibrium.

Five components are required for healthy cells. They are listed here along with a few illustrations, including important factors under each category.

Cell Environment (Internal and External)

- Internal temperature is 98.6 degrees F for most people; 104-106 F are damaging.
- pH levels: Cells operate best from a pH of 7.0-7.3 (cancer cells cannot live in a pH of 6.5 or above).
- Stressors for cells include drugs, poisons, alcohol, and nicotine.
- Pure water is required in generous amounts (six to eight glasses a day, minimum).
- Oxygen must be present for cells to function.
- The blood must be filled with nutrients.

Cell Protection

- The skin filters out poisons.
- All mucous membranes protect cells from undesirable substances.
- Friendly bacteria in the intestines produce certain important nutrients.
- Tear glands keep eyeballs moist.
- Immune system components fight for us.
- Antibodies destroy disease and toxins.

Cell Exercise

- Exercise is required to empty cell waste.
- Exercise helps bones retain calcium.
- Bacteria, viruses, and other foreign matter can be removed by exercise.
- Exercise eliminates tiredness and lethargy due to poisons in the cell.

Positive Mental Attitude

- Healthy cells require a healthy mind.
- Cell damage results from emotions of resentment, hate, jealousy, fear, grief, or unforgiveness.
- Peace, joy, laughter, harmony, love, and happiness are the results of a positive mental attitude.

Cell Food

- Healthy cells require healthy foods.

THE POWER OF PURE WATER

The presence or absence of sufficient amounts of pure water greatly influences cell health. Body fluids carry oxygen and nutrients to the cells and carbon dioxide and waste away from them. The fluids must circulate to pick up fresh supplies and eliminate the wastes. Water plays a vital role in this process. We need water for the production of hormones, enzymes, digestive juices, interstitial fluid, and many other cell activities. Cells depend upon extra cellular fluid around them to carry oxygen from the lungs and other tissues.

Most Americans drink inadequate amounts of water for optimal cell functioning. As a rule, you should drink a minimum of six to eight glasses of water (sixty to eighty ounces) each day. If you exercise regularly, it is crucial to replace fluid loss (rehydrate) by drinking even more water. And we are talking about *water,* not just liquids of *any* kind. Soft drinks and coffee, for example, are *not* healthy substitutes.

A Final Thought

As we conclude this chapter, let me leave you with a final thought: Cells are perfectly capable of living, growing, reproducing, and performing their special functions as long as the blood, muscles, organs, glands, and body fluids bring them the proper concentrations of oxygen, glucose, vitamins, minerals, amino acids, and fatty substances required by our body's internal environment.

When choosing fuel for those cells, lean toward the natural foods that God has provided. They are best for building or maintaining excellent cell health. Choosing them is the very best way to build and maintain an optimal state of cell health and to care for our bodies in the way that God designed.

TEN

Special Fitness Challenges for Men and Women

DON OTIS

If you are experiencing a middle-age malaise, then you should examine your fitness level and eating habits to see whether you are destroying your vital energies.

—TIM LaHAYE

Moses was eighty years old when God called him out of shepherding to begin his life's most important task. Today, that would be fifteen years after many of us retire! The Bible doesn't mention Joshua's age when he took over Moses' duties, but he must have been even older; the rest of the Israelites died before they entered the Promised Land. In nearly every Sunday school class, children learn about God's promise to an aged Abraham. He was about one hundred years old when Isaac was born; his wife, Sarah, was ninety! The Bible is full of examples of men and women of *all* ages whom God used for His strategic purposes. God does not care about a person's race, age, gender, or skills when He calls them to service. He cares only about their willingness to be obedient to His call.

In the twenty-first century, God continues to call people to accomplish His purposes. Each of us has a different call centered on the same theme—to make God's will and purposes known on earth. This, of course, includes sharing the good news about redemption through Jesus Christ. To fulfill God's mandate requires that we have the energy, stamina, strength, mental capacity, and desire to carry out His will. Sadly, this is not always the case with some Christians. Instead, we are often tired, out of shape, or uninterested in doing the work of the kingdom. If we are not available—no matter what the reason—God will find someone who is. That is His way.

This book has not been about fitness for fitness's sake. Rather, it is about taking care of the temple God has given each of us. While our Creator has endowed us with very special gifts and calling, He has also made each of us physically unique. (Wouldn't the world be boring if we all looked the same?) No one, not even the best athlete in the world, can excel at everything. Can you remember when basketball great Michael Jordan took a year or two off from playing for the world champion Chicago Bulls basketball team to try baseball? His attempt was a dismal failure. All of us have a unique range of talents, interests, and physical attributes.

Some of those different physical and emotional attributes divide along gender lines. Men and women are different. God has made us different. It is part of His design. Different doesn't mean better or worse; it just means different. There are, of course, important similarities between men and women. Many kinds of cancer, heart disease, and obesity do not discriminate based on a person's sex or race. Yet it is no secret that, on average, women live longer than men. While the life expectancy of a baby born in the United States is seventy-seven, women tend to outlive men by five or six years. And for every one hundred women over sixty-five, there are only seventy-seven men.[1] Although this gap is expected to decrease in the next several decades, it remains a sociological reality that influences healthcare, retirement, and family issues.

This chapter examines the major physical differences that men and women face after forty. Of course, a man who has just entered his forties is dealing with different issues than a man entering retirement. But we will look at the major challenges men and women face in their quest to remain healthy at midlife and beyond.

Mental Calisthenics: Protecting Your Brain

Fifty-six percent of Baby Boomers are worried about developing Alzheimer's, a disease that destroys a person's mental capacities.[2] God's Word tells us to love the Lord with all our heart, soul, and mind (see Matthew 22:37). We love God by using the minds He has given us, by acknowledging Him with our intellect as well as with our emotions. Use seems to be a factor in keeping our brains healthy, just as use is a factor in keeping our bodies fit. The good news is that a drastic mental decline is not inevitable as we get older. However, definite changes do take place. For example, abstract reasoning begins to fade.

There are undoubtedly genetic and environmental factors that play a role in our mental capacities as we age. This does not mean there is nothing we can do to exercise our brains. In a longitudinal study looking at the factors that make up healthy mental processing, researchers found that those who have an above-average level of education, a complex and stimulating lifestyle, and who are married to a smart spouse are most likely to have strong mental functions at an older age. Conversely, rigid adherence to routine and low satisfaction with life negatively affect the brain. Likewise, idle minds tend to decay faster than those engaged in stimulating mental activities and new experiences. Hard-driving personality types who always insist on doing things their way are more susceptible to mental decline later in life. Those who are willing to try new things or to improvise generally have more mental acuity later.

While lifestyle and personality play a role in maintaining a healthy brain, exercise and diet are also crucial factors. Overeating, inactivity, and stress show up as predictors for physical and mental decay. Healthier brains are those that get more oxygen-rich blood flowing to them through exercise.

The logical question that arises is whether we can do anything to bolster our chances of staying mentally and physically sound. We already know the answer to the "physical" part of the question. Now, however, let's look at the mental aspects.

AT MIDDLE AGE

- *Develop expertise.* High levels of thought prime the brain, and often-used knowledge is best remembered.
- *Save more.* People with greater financial resources can treat themselves to mind-nourishing experiences such as travel and cultural events.
- *Achieve your major life goals now.* Those who head into retirement unfulfilled fare worse than those at peace with their accomplishments.
- *Enjoy the bustle.* The brain thrives on challenges, like many

of the complications that arise from midlife. But don't get overanxious; stress hormones may hurt the brain.

- *Avoid burnout.* Burnout often leads to withdrawal. Once the mind has slowed down, it's tough to get back up to speed.

AFTER AGE SIXTY-FIVE

- *Seek new horizons.* Novel experiences keep the mind limber. Resist the temptation to settle into a comfortable routine.
- *Engage the world.* Do things you believe make a difference in life. People who don't feel a sense of purpose tend to disengage from life and lose faculties sooner.
- *Take a daily walk* (exercise regularly). This can increase your score on intelligence tests.
- *Keep control.* A sense of helplessness leads to mental apathy and deterioration.

As a Christian, I would add the importance of prayer, meditation on God's Word, a sense of humor, and outreach to these lists. People who reach out to others in need (which Christ tells us to do) find a sense of peace and purpose in their lives. If retirement is simply a vehicle for personal relaxation, the mind and spirit will not be engaged beyond self-interest.

How Old Is Old?

It is no secret that as we get older we tend to define *old* as "someone who is older than we are." When asked, "At what age do you think someone becomes middle-aged?" nearly two-thirds of those surveyed said fifty years old or higher.[3] Chronological age is no longer the best description of age. You know what I mean when you see someone the same age as you who has lived a rough life. Perhaps they have been substance abusers or they neglected exercise or eating healthfully. They look tired, drawn, or hardened. Sin and abuse cause us to age faster. Proverbs says, "The fear of the LORD adds length to life, but the years of the wicked are cut short" (10:27). This biblical principle is proven at high school reunions every year!

But are there ways to slow the aging process? The answer is a definite yes. Here are a few suggestions:

- Explore mental and physical boundaries.
- Remain physically active.
- Maintain muscle strength.
- Control your lifestyle and habits (choose to live in a healthy way).
- Keep socially active.
- Nurture your spiritual life (tithe, pray, fast, meditate, learn).
- Stay optimistic, smile, laugh.
- Don't accept chronological age as a barrier. Physiological age is a better predicator of age.
- See your doctor on a regular basis.

Now we turn our attention to the specific issues related to men and women as they get older. First we start with health and fitness as it relates to men over forty.

Special Health and Fitness Issues for Men

Women aren't the only ones who fight the image of the perfect body. Men's magazines push better sex, stronger muscles, and perfect abs. The pictures are as unrealistic for middle-aged and older men as are the near-anorexic twenty-something women glaring from the covers of women's magazines. The truth is, most men will never look like the men in the fitness magazines. As men reach their forties, this can become a depressing reality. For some, it can be the catalyst for a midlife crisis.

Just what exactly happens to men as they get older? How does the body change? For most of us, we already know the answers. By the time we reach our forties, fifties, sixties, and beyond, we realize that we are probably not going to become elite athletes. Instead, middle age is the time most men make mental and physical adjustments, revising exercise routines and expectations.

Some medical experts refer to "male menopause." Perhaps this is a bad description. It implies that there are clear biological markers (as there are in women) for the changes that take place in men. Women's biological changes are definable. The changes that occur in men are nebulous. Here are some of the changes middle-aged men can expect.

- Between the ages of twenty-five and seventy-five, body fat nearly doubles, especially in muscles and organs.
- Aerobic endurance decreases. The capacity of a seventy-year-old is only half that of a twenty-year-old. The body begins to lose its ability to deliver oxygen.
- Maximal heart rate decreases. This makes it more difficult for the heart to respond efficiently to physical exertion.
- The brain's ability to store and retrieve information declines slightly but steadily.
- By age fifty there is a noticeable loss of night vision and close-in focus (farsightedness) due to thickening of the lenses.
- The number of hair follicles on the scalp decreases, and the hair that is left grows at a slower rate.

- Eardrums thicken and the ear canal atrophies, making pure tones and high frequencies harder to hear.
- The chest wall stiffens, increasing the work load on respiratory muscles.
- Muscles get smaller and weaker.
- Bone loss occurs at individual rates.
- Sex drive declines due to lower levels of sex hormones. The number of orgasms decreases from an average of 2.3 per week in the thirties to 1.6 in the forties, 1.0 in the fifties, 0.6 in the sixties, and 0.4 in the seventies.[4]

These markers, which begin at middle age, lead to depression in some men. This is understandable. Midlife is often the time men start to recognize their own mortality. It is when older children are heading off to college and aging parents need extra help or care. The stress from family, job, marriage, and finances—coupled with physical and sexual decline—can lead to the so-called midlife crisis.

NAVIGATING MIDLIFE ISSUES

At midlife some men feel the need to buy a Harley-Davidson, climb the Alps, or go to extremes to make themselves attractive to the opposite sex (often falling for younger women). They are seeking to reclaim some of their childhood or to prove that they can still perform at a certain level. As a result, some men succumb to temptations during this time of life. A man may leave his wife for a younger woman only to find that his unhappiness remains. Male midlife crises are often characterized by irrational decision making, desperation, or catastrophe. Why does this happen?

First, it is at this point in our lives when many of us start to realize we have not achieved our dreams. We may spend time looking at how we could have lived our lives differently. We all have regrets about some decision or lack of decision that could or should have been made. But God loves us in spite of our imperfections and wants to build us into true models of character. We may never become standout quarterbacks or chief executive officers for Fortune 500 companies, but we can be standout role models to our families, wives, or communities. That's really all God asks from us—to be a light and example of Him wherever we are.

A second issue men face in midlife is a major restructuring of family. Children are no longer a diversion; soccer games, baseball, fishing, or school activities no longer demand our time. All of a sudden, men find themselves alone, perhaps forced to deal with marital relationship issues for the first time in their lives. Of course, this can be a positive time to reflect and move into a new phase of life. For some men, however, it is stressful, new, lonely, and uncomfortable. Christian men need to get plugged in with other men— going beyond PromiseKeepers' gatherings or single special events. They need true companionship in which they can share openly, ask questions, and form lasting bonds. In his book *Old Man, New Man,* Stephen Strang writes, "I believe most men want close friends in spite of the fact that as a group men tend to process things more individually than women might. Even though much of a man's life is spent projecting a confident, strong, handle-what-comes image of himself and others, deep down inside he doesn't like being an island."[5]

A third, and perhaps the most obvious, influence in men at midlife is the physical changes we discussed earlier. If a man has neglected his health, midlife is the time he starts paying the piper. Although men will feel the typical results of aging—aches and pains, joint stiffness, and shortness of breath—the big issues such as heart disease and cancer are suddenly foremost in their thinking. These physical fears coupled with a waning sex drive, baldness, weight gain, and muscle loss can lead a man to make drastic (though not always bad) changes.

Here are some practical suggestions for men to avoid or minimize a crisis in their midlife years.

- Get in shape—or stay in shape—physically.
- Eat right.
- Get plenty of rest.
- Maintain close family relationships.
- Don't hold grudges.
- Don't neglect your marriage.
- Start or join a men's small group for fellowship and accountability.
- Develop or maintain healthy male friendships.
- If you are married, develop and maintain lasting friendships with other couples.
- Direct or redirect efforts to serve others (outreach).
- Revise your expectations for yourself and others.
- Set realistic goals for the future (don't live in the past).
- Express thankfulness to God and others.
- Learn to have fun and to laugh.
- Don't avoid medical checkups (see following list).

A MEDICAL CHECKLIST

There is an abundance of information about medical issues that affect men. Still, there are several tests that every man over forty needs to know about. Depending on your family history and health, you may need additional tests. Don't put off having these simple tests done. More important, don't assume that because you have been healthy your entire life you don't need the tests at this point in your life.

- blood pressure (every one to two years) to control hypertension and prevent complications from kidney or heart failure
- weight and height to detect hypertension or diabetes
- skin exam (every one to three years) to look for melanoma
- neck exam (detects thyroid cancer)
- heart exam (every one to three years) to detect murmurs
- abdominal exam (every one to three years) to detect aortic aneurysm and liver or spleen enlargement
- lymph node exam (every one to three years) to check for lymphoma
- groin exam (every one to three years) to check for inguinal hernia
- testicular exam (every one to three years) to detect tumors
- prostate exam (annually for men over fifty-five) to detect nodules that may require further testing for prostate cancer[6]

It is worth noting that for men who run, the incidence of prostate problems is 25 percent lower than it is for those who are sedentary.[7] And in recent studies, men who ate ten or more servings of tomato products a week have a 45 percent lower chance of developing prostate cancer.[8] These encouraging, preventive measures are a compelling reason to maintain exercise and adjust eating habits.

Although most men are becoming more aware of the risk factors for certain kinds of male-related diseases such as prostate cancer, many are reluctant to see a doctor unless they experience a problem. But we don't wait until our car engine seizes up before we schedule an oil change. So why do we wait to see a doctor until we have difficulty urinating or notice a suspicious swelling? Make it a point to visit your physician regularly and ask about the appropriate exams for your age group.

Physical examinations are not the only tests men should have. Here are a few laboratory tests that men over forty need to include in their overall health plan:

- blood count to test for anemia and leukemia and to check platelet counts
- urinalysis to look for the presence of glucose, protein, blood cells, bacteria, and crystals
- chemical profile: total cholesterol (coronary disease risk factor), HDL cholesterol (good cholesterol), LDL cholesterol (bad cholesterol), and triglycerides (fatty acids)
- other chemical analyses, including those that check blood nitrogen, liver function, uric acid, and calcium

Cholesterol tests are cheap, relatively painless, and they provide immediate results. Because cholesterol is such a popular concern, let me explain what each of the above-mentioned measures means and why each is important.

Our bodies need cholesterol to function properly. Yet if we have too much in our blood, it can clog our arteries and lead to a heart attack. Exercise and prudent eating habits can keep your cholesterol level where it is supposed to be (a desirable level is less than 200 mg/dL).

HDL, or good cholesterol, helps clear excess cholesterol from the arteries. The higher the number, the better. A good level is anything more than 35 mg/dL.

LDL, or bad cholesterol, contributes to the buildup of deposits on arterial walls. An LDL level of less than 130 mg/dL is best.

Triglycerides are composed of fatty acids and glycerol (which provides energy for the body). Small amounts are always circulating in the blood, and these increase after a meal. If your body processes fat efficiently, the level of triglycerides will decrease. The optimal measurements are less than 126 mg/dL (fasting) and less than 160 mg/dL (nonfasting).

Special Health and Fitness Issues for Women

Despite the headlines in women's magazines, a perfect body is not only a myth, it is an obsession that Western culture ceaselessly perpetuates. For the Christian woman, health should be a matter of taking care of the vessel God has given her. No more, no less. A constant striving for perfection and youth will likely leave the woman at midlife discouraged, depressed, and unable to fight her way out of societal expectations. It is simplistic to say Christian women need to reject this unrealistic stereotyping, but that's exactly what needs to happen.

There are other unfortunate aging issues in American culture that affect women. As women age, their bodies go through definitive changes that are both similar to and unique from men. In this section, we will concentrate on those areas that are most age-specific to women over forty.

- More than 25 percent of all women develop osteoporosis, or thinning of the bones, within ten to fifteen years of menopause.
- More than a third of women thirty to forty-nine are overweight. After menopause, more than 50 percent of all women are overweight (tripling the risk for heart disease and stroke).[9]
- Basal metabolic rate (BMR) decreases. This is the rate at

which your body consumes energy while you are awake. The single most important factor in your BMR is the amount of your lean body tissue (something that can be controlled by exercise and muscle building).

- Starting at age forty, women lose about one-third of a pound of muscle every year (and gain about that much body fat). Strength training can help this imbalance.
- Difficulty with balance begins in midlife and gradually worsens as women reach their seventies. Again, strength training can minimize this.
- Flexibility in shoulders, knees, ankles, and hips decreases.
- Loss of libido occurs, particularly after menopause. In addition, vaginal dryness caused by a reduction of estrogen levels can cause pain or discomfort during intercourse.
- Urinary irritations increase, caused by tissue thinning near the urethra. This makes the urinary tract more susceptible to irritation and infection.
- Breast cancer kills 44,000 women every year. Exercising seven or more hours a week can cut your risk by 20 percent.[10]
- Heart disease is the number-one killer of women over fifty. Each year, 500,000 women die of cardiovascular disease, which is largely preventable through exercise and diet.[11]

A MEDICAL CHECKLIST

Most women, by the time they reach their midlife years, have experienced protracted stress. The expectations placed on them are enormous, and it is little wonder more don't succumb to physical or mental distress. In many instances they have been accustomed to addressing the immediate needs of their families while spending very little time looking after themselves. The good news is that God has created our bodies to "throw off" the effects of most levels of stress through physical exertion or exercise. Women who exercise feel calmer and more relaxed. Those who remain physically active find their midlife and senior years to be enormously satisfying. The reason? They have more energy to engage in physically challenging activities or to chase grandkids around. They also experience fewer age-related health problems than those who have remained sedentary. Of course, part of staying healthy is getting regular checkups. All women over forty should have the following tests to ensure lasting health:

- blood pressure to check for hypertension
- weight and height (factors in diabetes and osteoporosis)
- skin exam to detect cancers like melanoma
- neck exam to check for thyroid cancer
- breast exam to detect lumps
- heart exam to detect murmurs and infection of the heart valve
- abdominal exam to detect liver or spleen enlargement
- lymph node exam to detect lymphoma

It is also recommended that all women between forty and forty-nine have a mammogram every two years; after fifty, it should be done annually.

THE GREAT HORMONE DEBATE

Should women use hormone replacement therapy (HRT)? Although this is not a major focus of this book, it is an issue for women struggling with weight problems, tiredness, sleeplessness, or those trying to accelerate postoperative healing.

By the time women reach middle age, their weight steadily

climbs, resulting in an average weight gain of twelve pounds between thirty-five and fifty. This gain can be directly correlated to the decline in estrogen levels and a woman's move toward menopause. Her metabolism simply cannot burn the calories it did when she was younger.[12]

Symptoms most commonly associated with lack of estrogen are mood swings, hot flashes, memory loss, insomnia, and increased risk of osteoporosis. As a result, estrogen is one of the hormones commonly used in HRT. Proponents of estrogen replacement argue that life expectancy increases and it helps prevent osteoporosis and heart disease in postmenopausal women. There are, however, some side effects that cannot be ignored. These include cramping, breast pain (and possibly risk of breast cancer), and weight gain.

Here is a very brief look at three other natural hormones and their benefits and risks to women.

Testosterone declines most notably in men after forty and women after fifty. It can improve mood and increase the sex drive in both men and women as they age. The side effects include a possible decrease in HDL cholesterol and an increase in LDL cholesterol, increasing the risk for stroke or heart disease.

Human growth hormone can cause a shift in the body's metabolism, creating more muscle and less fat. It also helps healing in surgical patients and improves deep sleep. However, it may lead to carpal tunnel syndrome, diabetes-like symptoms, and breast tenderness.

Melatonin declines at about age forty. It helps insomnia in adults and may boost the immune system for fighting cancer. The side effects are grogginess and depression in some people.[13]

Fearfully and Wonderfully Made

No matter what your age or gender, the Bible tells us that God made us special and unique. No other part of His creation is like the human machine. This is surely something to celebrate. We are not accidental by-products of random forces; instead Christians recognize the magnificence of intelligent design in the human body.

God's ways are not arbitrary in the design of our bodies any more than they are in the interest He takes in our daily lives. He cares for us. In turn, we should care for the beauty and function He has created in our physical beings. By caring for God's most precious of creations—our bodies—we honor Him.

Vitamins and Minerals: What We Need, Why We Need Them

JUDY LINDBERG MCFARLAND

The whole idea of a vitamin is a paradox and difficult to digest. Everybody knows that things we eat can make us sick, but it seems utterly senseless to say that something which we have not eaten could make us sick. And this is exactly what a vitamin is: a substance which makes us sick and even die by not eating it.

—ALBERT SZENT-GYORGI, M.D., PH.D.[1]

The late Albert Szent-Gyorgi was a brilliant researcher who received the Nobel Prize in physiology and medicine, as well as the Albert Lasker Prize for his theory of muscle contraction. I believe that his classic statement above truly reflects the great importance of vitamins. If we do not obtain the vitamins or minerals we need from our food supply or in supplement form, we can become sick and even die.

Many people are realizing that the average American diet is far from adequate and actually causes some of the diseases we face today, such as heart disease, many forms of cancer, diabetes, osteoporosis, and arthritis.

Other conditions such as allergies, premature aging, obesity, chronic fatigue, impotence, and birth defects can also be directly related to nutritional imbalances in our bodies. Deficiencies of certain vitamins and minerals can be involved in the death of millions of Americans annually. In order to recognize and correct our habits, it's important to learn what vitamins and minerals are and why we need them.

Vitamins

A vitamin is a group of organic compounds that, in very small amounts, are essential for normal growth, development, and metabolism. With a few exceptions, they cannot be synthesized or made in the body and must be supplied by the diet. Vitamins are produced by living material, such as plants and animals, while minerals come from the soil. Lack of a sufficient quantity of any vitamin produces specific deficiency diseases. In fact, if a substance does not produce a deficiency symptom when it is removed from the diet, it is not considered a vitamin.

Each vitamin functions in many diverse roles and always with other essential nutrients. Vitamins participate in a variety of life-building processes, including the formation and maintenance of blood cells, hormones, all the cells and tissues of the body, and even the creation of our genetic material.

Vitamins are not used as sources of energy as some believe. They contain no calories, and they cannot make you fat. They are used to form enzymes that are biologic catalysts in many metabolic reactions within the body. Several vitamins help convert the calories in carbohydrates, protein, and fat into usable energy for the body. In other words, vitamins are not the fuel, but they are the ignition switch that sparks the fuel and keeps the engine running. When vitamins are not present in sufficient quantity, metabolism ceases or is impaired.

When you perspire, take diuretic drugs (such as high-blood-pressure medication), or have diarrhea, you lose an abnormal amount of water-soluble vitamins. Stress and exertion also deplete the body of these valuable nutrients. Actually, our supply of these vitamins is constantly being diminished by the activity of our own bodies. Therefore, if we are to maintain even reasonably good health, these vitamins have to be replaced on a routine basis.

I am often asked if we really need to take vitamin and mineral supplements. The good news is that I hear this question less today than several years ago; the general public is becoming much more informed about the need for vitamins and minerals. Still, a great many people seem to believe that they can get all their daily requirements for vitamins and minerals from a "well-balanced diet" without taking additional supplements. The diet we tend to think about as being well balanced is one that came from our nation's agricultural heritage. Our great-grandparents came from the farm, where they performed hard physical labor all day and consumed between 4,000 and 5,000 calories per day. They got their milk right from the cow and their fruits and vegetables from the garden. They ground their own whole grains and ate five or six times a day. They did not need vitamin or mineral supplements because they received enough of these nutrients from the large amounts of natural and fresh foods they consumed.

Most of us today cannot consume those large amounts of natural and fresh foods as our ancestors did. We don't do as much physical labor so we cannot burn the extra calories. The food we eat today varies considerably in the amount of nutrients it contains, the way it is grown, the chemicals sprayed on it, how it is processed, and in the way we store or prepare it in our kitchens.

The United States Department of Agriculture has stated that as many as one out of every two Americans is not getting the minimum RDA (Recommended Dietary Allowance) as the result of his or her current diet. Even though these guidelines reflect a minimal level, one-half of our population falls below the minimum.[2] The studies that follow reflect this deficiency.

- *Time* magazine has reported that about only 9 percent of Americans consume five servings a day of fruit and vegetables, according to the National Center for Health Statistics.

- A USDA survey of 21,500 people over a three-day period showed that not one of them consumed 100 percent of the RDA for ten nutrients.

- Surveys have shown that on the average an elderly person takes between six and nine prescription drugs a day. Many of these drugs rob the body of vitamins and minerals in a variety of ways, such as: increasing urinary excretion, blocking absorption, binding to nutrients and deactivating them, destroying nutrients, causing nutrients to be used up more rapidly, and increasing loss of nutrients in the stool.[3]

One of the most intelligent decisions a person can make is to take vitamin and mineral supplements daily. When clients tell me they cannot afford vitamins, I tell them our Lindberg Vitamin and Mineral packets cost less than a cup of coffee or a soft drink. I explain to them *they cannot afford NOT to take them!* Vitamins and minerals are among the best anti-aging, health-building insurance policies.

I also reassure people that vitamins are safe and effective. Studies show that vitamins are 2,500 times safer than drugs. Doctors who recognize the benefits of vitamin therapy are recommending them to overcome high cholesterol, reduce cancer risk, and prevent or relieve many chronic health problems.[4]

Julian Whitaker, M.D., writes, "According to detailed analysis of all available data, there are over ten million adverse reactions yearly from FDA-approved over-the-counter and prescription drugs. We are not talking about mild nausea or headaches. Between 60,000 and 149,000 people per year die from adverse drug reactions, according to the *Journal of the American Medical Association.* Each year, more Americans die after taking prescription drugs than died in the entire Vietnam War. This constitutes a real public health issue."[5]

Many scientists champion the safety of vitamins even when taken in large amounts. Abram Hoffer, M.D., Ph.D., writes in the *Journal of Orthomolecular Medicine*: "Vitamins which are safe even in large doses have not been acceptable to the medical profession, and their negative side effects have been consistently exaggerated and over-emphasized without there being any scientific evidence that these side effects are real."[6]

Research continues to show the benefits, not the dangers of vitamins.

Minerals

Just as with vitamins, never underestimate the importance of minerals to your total well-being. People often think of minerals as relating only to teeth and bones, but minerals also preserve the vigor of the heart and brain, as well as the muscles and the entire nervous system. About 5 percent of your total body weight is mineral matter. Minerals are found in your bones, teeth, nerve cells, muscles, soft tissues, and blood.

Minerals are important in the production of hormones and enzymes, in the creation of antibodies, and in keeping the blood and tissue fluids from becoming either too acidic or too alkaline. Some minerals, such as sodium, potassium, and calcium, have electrical charges that act as a magnet to attract other electrically charged substances to form complex molecules, conduct electrical impulses along nerves, or transport substances in and out of the cells. In the blood and other fluids, minerals regulate the fluid pressure between cells and the blood. Minerals also bind to proteins and other organic substances and are found in red blood cells, all cell membranes, hormones, and enzymes, the catalysts of all bodily processes.[7]

Mineral or trace-element deficiencies occur much more often than vitamin deficiencies. Those at increased risk for mineral deficiencies are people who eat low-calorie diets; the elderly; pregnant women; vegetarians; those who take certain drugs, including diuretics; and those living in areas where the soil has been depleted of certain minerals.

Vitamins are usually present in foods in similar amounts around the world, but this is not true for minerals. Geologic conditions make certain areas rich in minerals, while the soil in other areas of the world is scarce in minerals.

Minerals can work together or against each other. Some compete for absorption. When this happens, a large intake of one mineral can actually produce a deficiency of another. This is especially true of the trace minerals iron, zinc, and copper. Some minerals can enhance the absorption and use of other minerals, as in the case of calcium, magnesium, and phosphorous, which all work together well.

Conclusion

New information about various vitamins, minerals, and antioxidants is constantly reported in the news. It is one of the most exciting and rapidly growing fields of research. I encourage you to stay abreast of the information about these substances and add them to your nutritional program. They may very well be the foremost key to your staying in excellent health.[8]

Notes

Introduction

1. "Strength Training When You're 50+," *IDEA: The Health & Fitness Source,* 2000. For more information, contact 1-800-999-4332.
2. Virginia Stem Owens, "The Fatted Faithful," *Christianity Today,* 11 January 1999, 70-2.
3. Katherine Webster, "Study: Obesity Can Shorten Lifespan," Associated Press, 7 October 1999.
4. Don Colbert, M.D., *What You Don't Know May Be Killing You* (Lake Mary, Fla.: Siloam Press, 2000), 128.
5. "Americans urged to do something—anything," *Spokane (Wash.) Spokesman-Review,* 26 January 2000, A5.
6. "Strong Faith Linked to Better Health," Charisma News Service, 20 July 1999.
7. Alisa Bauman, "Running on Faith," *Runner's World,* June 1999, 86.
8. Kelly McBride, "The Power of Prayer," *Spokane (Wash.) Spokesman-Review,* 23 May 1999, F1.
9. Melissa August, et al., "Numbers," *Time,* 25 October 1999, 48.
10. Usha Lee McFarling, "Americans fighting battle of the bulge," *Spokane (Wash.) Spokesman-Review,* 4 November 1999, A2.

Chapter One

1. Vickie and Jayme Farris, *A Mom Just Like You* (Sisters, Ore.: Loyal Publishing, 2000), 210.

2. Bob Wischnia and Joe Kita, "Run Healthy Forever," *Runner's World,* January 2000, 46.

3. James Sturz, "The Rest of Your Life," *Men's Health,* July/August 1997, 74.

4. *Runner's World,* October 2000, 22.

CHAPTER TWO

1. Joseph B. Verrengia, "Study: Walks Help Boost Memory," Associated Press, 28 July 1999.

2. Alisa Bauman, "Running Lifts Depression," *Runner's World,* March 2000, 19.

3. Michele Stanten, "Do This Before You Indulge," *Prevention,* July 1999, 72.

4. Megan Othersen Gorman, "Just for Kicks," *Runner's World,* October 1999, 50.

CHAPTER THREE

1. W. Terry Whalin, "The Rewards of a Disciplined Life," 8 September 2000, http://www.christianity.com.

2. "Rev Up Your Metabolism," *Prevention,* July 1998, 100.

CHAPTER FOUR

1. Dave Carpenter, "Health Clubs Expect Senior Boom," Associated Press, 19 October 1999.

2. Eileen Portz-Shovlin, "The Human Race," *Runner's World,* February 2000, 85.

3. Bob Wischnia and Joe Kita, "Run Healthy Forever," *Runner's World,* January 2000, 47.

4. Heather Lalley, "Exercise Evangelist," *Spokane (Wash.) Spokesman-Review,* 22 October 1999.

5. Jacqui Podzius Cook, "Study: Exercise Reduces Stroke Risk," Associated Press, 14 June 2000.
6. "Jog for Mental Health," Associated Press, 3 January 2000.
7. "You Can Prevent Osteoporosis," *Newsweek* Special Issue, spring/summer 1999, 61.
8. "Hopkins: Benefits of Exercise in the Elderly," Johns Hopkins University, 20 November 1997.
9. "Don't Take It Easy—Exercise!" National Institute on Aging, http://www.nih.gov/nia/health.
10. "Don't Take It Easy—Exercise!"
11. A. S. Leon, et al., "Leisure-Time Physical Activity Levels and Risk of Coronary Heart Disease and Death," *Journal of the American Medical Association* 258 (1987): 2388-95.

CHAPTER FIVE

1. Dr. Gregg Jantz, *21 Days to Eating Better* (Grand Rapids, Mich.: Zondervan, 1998).
2. Niloufar Motamed, "The Buddy System," *Women's Sports & Fitness,* September 2000, 21.

CHAPTER SIX

1. D. Menard and W. D. Stanish, "The Aging Athlete," *American Journal of Sports Medicine* 17, no. 2 (1989): 19.
2. P. H. Fentem, "ABC of Sports Medicine: Benefits of exercise in health and disease," *BMJ* 308 (1994): 1,291-5.
3. R. G. Ross, *Sports Medicine,* American Academy of Family Physicians Monograph 222 (1997).
4. Special Medical Reports, *American Family Physician* 54, no. 2 (August 1996).

5. R. Charles Bull, *Handbook of Sports Injuries* (New York: McGraw-Hill, 1999), 191.

6. Bull, *Handbook of Sports Injuries,* 183.

7. Bull, *Handbook of Sports Injuries,* 183.

8. Adapted from Robert E. Sallis and Ferdy Massimino, *Essentials of Sports Medicine* (St. Louis, Mo.: Mosby, 1997), 518; and R. G. Ross, *Sports Medicine,* 23.

9. John Wilkinson, *The Bible and Healing* (Grand Rapids, Mich.: Wm. B. Eerdman, 1998), 17.

CHAPTER SEVEN

1. Kathy Smith, "The Truth About Strength Training," *Los Angeles Times,* 11 January 1999, S4.

CHAPTER EIGHT

1. "Catching Up with…," *Runner's World,* February 2000, 15.

CHAPTER NINE

1. Dr. Michael Blumenkrantz, "Obesity: The World's Oldest Metabolic Disorder," http://www.quantumhcp.com/obesity.htm.

CHAPTER TEN

1. "The Age Boom," *The New York Times Magazine,* 9 March 1997, 39.

2. "Baby Boomers at Midlife," *Congressional Quarterly* 8 no. 28 (7 July 1998): 652.

3. "Baby Boomers at Midlife," 652.

4. Geoffrey Cowley, "Attention: Aging Men," *Newsweek,* 16 September 1996, 69-70.

5. Stephen Strang, *Old Man, New Man* (Lake Mary, Fla.: Creation House, 2000), 259.

6. Robert J. Weiss, et al., *40+ Guide to Good Health* (Yonkers, N.Y.: Consumers Union, 1993), 140-1.

7. Bob Wischnia and Joe Kita, "Run Healthy Forever," *Runner's World,* January 2000, 43.

8. Rick Chillot, "Men's Secret Fear," *Prevention,* July 1999, 124.

9. Miriam Nelson, Ph.D., and Sarah Wernick, *Strong Women Stay Slim* (New York: Bantam, 1998), 7.

10. Wischnia and Kita, "Run Healthy Forever," 42.

11. Karen Lee, A.R.N.P., "About Women's Health," http://www.womencare.com/facts.html.

12. Michele Meyer, "Outsmart Your Midlife Fat Cell," *Better Homes and Gardens,* May 2000, 278.

13. Benedict Carey, "Hooked on Youth," *Health,* November/December 1995, 74.

APPENDIX

1. Albert Szent-Gyorgi, M.D., Ph.D., "How New Understandings About the Biological Function of Ascorbic Acid May Profoundly Affect Our Life!" *Executive Health* (May 1978).

2. Gladys Lindberg and Judy McFarland, *Take Charge of Your Health* (San Francisco: Harper & Row, 1982), 181.

3. Karolyn A. Gazella, "Nutritional Supplements: Protecting the Core of American Health," *Health Counselor* 5.3: 27-31.

4. Paul Harvey, "Vitamins Are a 'Health Hazard'?" *Los Angeles Times Syndicate* 1992.

5. *Journal of the American Medical Association* 226 (1991): 2847-51.

6. Abram Hoffer, M.D., *Journal of Orthomolecular Medicine* 7 (first quarter 1992): 1.

7. Elizabeth Somer, *The Essential Guide to Vitamins and Minerals* (New York: Harper Perennial, 1992).

8. For the latest in vitamins, minerals, sports nutrition, and diet products contact Lindberg Nutrition, 3804 Sepulveda Blvd., Torrance, CA 90505, www.LindbergNutrition.com, or write: P.O. Box 3669, Torrance, CA 90510-3669 and ask for their mail order catalog–Nutrition Express (1-800-338-7979). This appendix was excerpted and edited with permission from Judy Lindberg McFarland, *Aging Without Growing Old* (Palos Verdes, Calif.: Western Front Publishing, 2000).

About the Contributors

Don S. Otis is the author of *Trickle-Down Morality* (Chosen Books) and *Teach Your Children Well* (Revell). Don is forty-four years old, has competed in triathlons throughout the western U.S., and has run in dozens of road races for more than twenty years. He has run the Sea of Galilee Marathon and climbed mountains on three continents. He lives with his wife, Susan, and their three sons in Sandpoint, Idaho.

Laurie Ellsworth is the author of *A Heart of Excellence* (Christian Publications-Horizon) and is a personal trainer and fitness educator. Laurie, who is forty years old, received her degree in kinesiology from the University of Illinois. She lives with her husband, Mike, and three children in Champaign, Illinois.

Gregory L. Jantz, Ph.D., holds a doctoral degree in counseling and health psychology and is the executive director of the Center for Counseling and Health Services headquartered in Edmonds, Washington. He is the author of eight books, including *Hope, Help and Healing for Eating Disorders* (Harold Shaw); *21 Days to Eating Better* (Zondervan); and *Losing Weight Permanently* (Harold Shaw). Gregory is forty-two years old and has cycled from Seattle to Portland every year for the past seven years. He competes in fun runs in the Northwest. He and his wife, LaFon, live in Seattle with their son, Gregg.

Tom Mason is vice president at Focus on the Family and former vice president of sales for General Motors in Europe and vice president of marketing for General Motors in Canada. Tom is a fifty-seven-year-old runner and skier. He has run in the Peachtree Road Race in Atlanta eighteen of the last nineteen years. He lives with his wife in Colorado Springs, Colorado.

Judy Lindberg McFarland is the owner of Nutrition Express and Lindberg Nutrition. She served as program chairman and president of the American Nutrition Society and has been a member of National Nutrition Foods Association. She holds a degree in nutrition from Pepperdine University and is the author of *Aging Without Growing Old*.

Jeff Mitchum is the founding pastor of Calvary Chapel in Point Loma, California. He has run the world-famous Ironman Triathlon in Hawaii and Ironman Switzerland three times. Jeff is a forty-two-year-old former All-American Triathlete who has run marathons in Boston, Los Angeles, Las Vegas, and Big Sur. Jeff runs, swims, cycles, and does strength training. He lives with his wife, Carolyn, in Encinitas, California.

Andrew M. Seddon, M.D., received his M.D. from the University of Maryland School of Medicine and now serves as staff physician at Deaconess Billings Clinic. Andrew is the author of *Imperial Legions* (Broadman & Holman) and *Red Plant Rising* (Crossway) and has written more than seventy articles on health, medicine, and medical ethics. He is forty-one years old and enjoys tennis and hiking in his hometown of Billings, Montana.

Mary Ruth Swope, Ph.D., is the author of *The Roots and Fruits of Fasting* and *Surviving the 20th Century Diet: Scientific Solutions to a Diet Gone Wrong* (Swope Enterprises). She earned her doctorate in administration from Columbia University and holds a master's degree in foods and nutrition from the University of North Carolina. She spent twenty years as the dean of the School of Economics at Eastern Illinois University. At eighty-two years old, Mary Ruth is an avid walker and founder of Barley Green. She resides in Avinger, Texas.

Maryanna Young is the president of Fitness Management Group, an agency specializing in the business management of professional athletes. Maryanna cofounded the Idaho Women's Fitness Celebration, an event with twenty thousand participants of all ages. She received her degree in exercise physiology and physical education from Oral Roberts University. She was voted Outstanding NCAA Student Athlete of the Year (specializing in five-thousand and ten-thousand meters) and received the President's Cup for her contribution to sports and the community. Maryanna runs, mountain bikes, and strength trains. She also plays basketball and tennis, and cross-country skis and hikes near her home in Boise, Idaho.

Printed in the United States
by Baker & Taylor Publisher Services